STOMA S

Redefining Life, One day at a Time

Shared Experience By;

JUDITH V. FENTON

TABLE OF CONTENT

INTRODUCTION 3

I: UNDERSTANDING OSTOMY SURGERY 9

PART 2: THE EMOTIONAL EXPERIENCE 19

PART 3: UNDERSTANDING YOUR STOMA 34

PART 4: MASTERING OSTOMY CARE 46

PART 5: NUTRITION AND DIETARY CHANGES 64

PART 6: LIFESTYLE ADJUSTMENTS AND DAILY LIFE 75

PART 7: RELATIONSHIP AND INTIMACY 97

PART 8: LONG-TERM HEALTH AND OSTOMY MAINTENANCE 106

Glossary of Terms 112

Common Medical Codes and Insurance Tips 114

List of National and International Ostomy Support Organization 116

Manucfacturers and Suppliers of Ostomy Products 118

INTRODUCTION

On that fateful day, my life shifted gears. The quiet hum of machinery, the antiseptic air of the hospital room, and the heaviness of the airborne air of doubt. As he spoke to me, my doctor held the key to my future. "They're suggesting an ostomy," he said. This was a word that didn't fit in my reality; it was strange and surreal. The idea of having an ostomy—a phrase that would soon reshape my whole existence—loomed large over me.

In the United States, more than 725,000 people live with an ostomy, a figure that grows internationally to about 3 million. Cancer, Crohn's disease, ulcerative colitis, and catastrophic injuries force tens of thousands of people to make the same choice I made every year. Many people experience the same emotions that I do when they consider a life with an ostomy: dread, bewilderment, and loss.

Ostomy is more than a medical illness; it's a transformative experience, and this book is here to help you through it. As someone who has been through this, I can attest that having an ostomy affects more than just your physical functioning; it also alters your viewpoint, relationships, and attitude on life. It requires you to face the delicate balance of sensitivity and strength, all while negotiating the various physical and emotional difficulties that come with it.

Why This Book is a Must-Read

There are lots of medical texts out there, full of facts and figures, but what is usually missing is the human element—the stories of people who have been through it, lived it, and emerged stronger. This book provides a blend of personal experience and practical advice, provided by someone who knows exactly what you're going through. I'll discuss the ups and downs, challenges I encountered, and surprising achievements along the way.

What distinguishes this work is its focus on real life. Living with an ostomy requires more than just surgery; it also involves adjusting to a new normal, learning to accept your body, and regaining confidence. Whether you're preparing for surgery, caring for someone with an ostomy, or just trying to make sense of your new situation, this book will assist you every step of the way. You'll find practical ideas, resources, and expert advice from healthcare professionals, all designed to help you live your best life post-ostomy.

The global need for ostomy knowledge and resources is increasing as awareness grows and stigmas are removed. This book is for everyone—whether you are one of the millions of people who live with an ostomy or you care about someone who does. It is a resource that not only educates but also inspires. From managing your new lifestyle to navigating relationships and work, I've compiled a list of things I wish I knew before embarking on this journey. My hope is that it may serve as a beacon of light for you, providing both comfort and empowerment as you walk your own path ahead.

Living with an ostomy is not the end; rather, it is the beginning. And this book is your guide as you embark on that journey, reminding you that life after an ostomy can be full of strength, joy, and hope.

An Introduction to Ostomy

When the regular route via the intestines or bladder is no longer functioning, waste (urine or stool) may be removed from the body through a surgically made hole in the abdomen called an ostomy. The waste is gathered in a bag or pouch that is exterior to the abdomen.

When illnesses, traumas, or congenital disorders impair the body's natural ability to eliminate waste, ostomies are life-saving procedures that restore physiological function. They are often required when severe disease or damage necessitates the bypassing or complete removal of portions of the digestive or urinary systems. Even while the thought of having an ostomy may seem daunting, it provides the possibility of a restored quality of life, free from the discomfort, suffering, or issues that made the procedure necessary.

An ostomy is used for the simple reason of enabling the body to expel waste when the regular pathway—via the intestines or bladder—is hampered.

Many individuals successfully live full, active lives with an ostomy, and with the right care and awareness, an ostomy may become simply another part of everyday life.

Colostomy, Ileostomy, and Urostomy:

Ostomies come in three main varieties, each based on the bodily parts involved. It's important to recognize the distinctions between them since they have different goals, need different surgical techniques, and require different aftercare.

Colostomy

A colon, or large intestine, ostomy, is referred to as a colostomy. This operation diverts waste from a part of the colon that is no longer working or has been removed.

A colostomy involves bringing a portion of the colon through the abdominal wall to form the stoma, or opening. This enables feces to gather in an external pouch after leaving the body via the stoma.
- Location: The positioning of the stoma might vary depending on which portion of the colon is impacted. The left, right, or center of the abdomen might be where it is positioned.
- Consistency of Output: Since colostomy stool originates in the large intestine, where water is reabsorbed from the waste, it is often more formed.
- Indications: Colostomies may be required in cases of diverticulitis, trauma, colorectal cancer, or inflammatory bowel disease (IBD).

Ileostomy

When the colon is injured or removed, an ileostomy is done on the ileum, the final segment of the small intestine.

An ileostomy is a procedure similar to a colostomy in which a stoma is created by bringing a part of the ileum through the abdominal wall. The colon is completely bypassed by waste from the small intestine.
- Location: The lower right side of the abdomen is where the stoma is usually found.

- Consistency of Output: The waste from an ileostomy is liquid or semi-formed and often includes digestive enzymes, which may irritate the skin surrounding the stoma. This is because the waste avoids the colon, which absorbs water.
- Indications: An ileostomy is often necessary for diseases such Crohn's disease, ulcerative colitis, familial polyposis, or colorectal cancer.

Urostomy

When the bladder is removed or bypassed, a urostomy is a surgical technique that directs urine out via a stoma instead of the bladder.

A tiny portion of the small intestine is utilized to establish a route that permits urine to travel from the kidneys to the stoma in a typical kind of urostomy known as an ileal conduit.

- Location: The lower abdomen's right side is usually where a urostomy stoma is located.
- Consistency of Output: A specifically made urostomy pouch collects urine that flows continuously from the stoma. Mucus may also be found in the urine, since a portion of the small intestine is utilized to build the conduit.
- Indications: A urostomy may be required in cases of bladder injuries, cancer, severe bladder disease, or congenital deformities.

Standard Causes of Ostomy Surgery

Ostomy surgery is often the final option when underlying medical issues significantly impair the body's capacity to eliminate waste products normally. The following are the most prevalent ailments that might result in ostomy surgery:

1. Cancer

One of the most frequent causes of ostomy surgery is cancer of the colon, rectum, bladder, or other digestive or urinary system organs.

- Colorectal Cancer: When malignant growths necessitate the removal of portions of the colon, a colostomy or ileostomy is often necessary.

- **Bladder Cancer:** If the bladder is removed to stop the cancer from spreading, a urostomy could be necessary.

In these situations, ostomy surgery may be permanent (when significant portions of the organ are removed) or temporary (to enable the colon to recover following surgery).

2. IBD, or inflammatory bowel disease

The digestive tract becomes chronically inflamed when an individual has an inflammatory bowel illness, such as Crohn's disease and ulcerative colitis. Complications such as intestinal blockage, severe inflammation, or even the breakdown of the intestinal wall may arise from these disorders over time.

- **Crohn's Disease:** This disorder may affect any region of the digestive system. An ileostomy could be required in extreme circumstances to circumvent damaged colon or small intestine sections
- **Ulcerative Colitis:** Exclusively affects the rectum and colon. A colectomy, or removal of the colon, may be necessary if medicine and other therapies are ineffective. This procedure often leaves patients with a lifelong ileostomy.

3. Diverticulitis

When tiny pouches (diverticula) develop in the colon and become inflamed or infected, it is known as Diverticulitis. In certain situations, these pouches might burst, leading to serious infection or abscesses. When this occurs, a colostomy—a portion of the colon removed—may be necessary.

Although diverticulitis is usually treated non-surgically, severe or repeated instances may need a temporary or permanent ostomy, especially if complications like fistulas or blockages develop.

4. Trauma

Serious abdominal injuries, including those from vehicle accidents, gunshot wounds, or knife wounds, may harm the bladder, intestines, or other organs to the point that an ostomy is necessary to channel waste while the body heals.

- Bowel Trauma: Trauma involving the small or large intestine may need a colostomy or ileostomy, either permanent or temporary.
- Bladder Trauma: A urostomy can be required if the bladder is damaged or has to be evacuated.

5. Hereditary Disorders

Some congenital abnormalities need ostomy surgery soon after birth or later in life because they impair the normal development of the urine or digestive systems. As examples, consider:

- Hirschsprung's Disease: A disorder where nerve cells in the colon are absent, leading to severe constipation or obstructions. It's possible that children with this illness may need an ileostomy or colostomy
- Bladder Exstrophy: A disorder in which the bladder is positioned outside the body or is malformed. Urinary function management may need a urostomy.

A vital first step in exploring the world of ostomies is understanding these fundamentals.

Part 1: Understanding Ostomy Surgery

Ostomy surgery might seem intimidating at first, but knowing the procedure step by step helps to demystify it and prepares you both psychologically and physically for the experience.

What Happens During Surgery: A Step-by-Step Guide

The exact technique for constructing an ostomy varies according to the kind of ostomy being done (colostomy, ileostomy, or urostomy). While the specifics of each form of ostomy vary somewhat, the general procedure follows a similar path:

- Pre-Surgery Preparation: Before surgery, you will be given general anesthesia, which will keep you sleeping and numb throughout the procedure. The surgical team will disinfect the region where the stoma will be put and make sure everything is prepared. For others, the scariest aspect is sitting in the antiseptic surroundings while hearing equipment beep. I recall feeling as if my life was in limbo, not exactly the person I was before the operation, but not quite the person I would become thereafter.
- Creating the Stoma: The surgeon creates an incision in the belly, usually on the lower left or right side, depending on the kind of ostomy. A little portion of the intestine (or, in the case of a urostomy, a portion of the urinary system) is dragged through the abdominal wall to form the stoma—a small, circular orifice on the skin's surface.

- The stoma permits waste to escape your body and collect in an external pouch.
- Resection and Bypass: Certain conditions, such as cancer, inflammatory bowel disease, or injury, may need the removal of parts of the colon or small intestine. An ileostomy will remove the small intestine, whereas a colostomy will remove the large intestine. The surgeon will gently join the healthy piece of the intestine to the stoma, ensuring that it works correctly.
- Closing the Abdomen: After the stoma is established and functional, the surgical team will seal the incision with sutures or staples. A tiny drainage tube may also be placed to avoid fluid accumulation during recovery.
- Testing and Ensuring Functionality: The surgeon will test the stoma before completing the procedure to guarantee proper functioning. The procedure may include examining the stoma's output and ensuring there are no leaks or problems.
- Recovery Room: After surgery, you will be brought to a recovery room where medical professionals will watch you until the anesthetic wears off. For me, this was the moment when reality set in. As I awoke in the recovery room, I instantly felt for my stomach, feeling the pouch's unusual texture. It was an emotional moment, understanding that life would never be the same again but also respecting the courage required to get here.

The complete process usually lasts between two and four hours, depending on the complexity and kind of surgery. After that, you'll spend a few days in the hospital learning how to care for your stoma and adapting to your new life.

The Differences between Temporary and Permanent Ostomies

When contemplating ostomy surgery, it is critical to determine if the operation is temporary or permanent. Each has a distinct impact on your health, recuperation, and future lifestyle.

Temporary Ostomies

A temporary ostomy is often used to allow the intestines to recover after surgery or injury. For example, if you had surgery to remove a segment of your colon due to cancer or diverticulitis, you may need a temporary ostomy while the remaining portions recover. Once the healing process is complete, which normally takes a few months, a second operation may be done to reverse the ostomy and rejoin the intestine.

- Purpose: Allow the intestines to recover.
- Duration: Temporary ostomies are usually reversed between 3 to 12 months, depending on the disease.
- Common conditions include inflammatory bowel disease, intestinal blockage, and trauma.

Knowing that my ostomy was just temporary did not make the procedure any easier. There was still terror, an overpowering feeling of loss, and unfamiliarity with my own body. However, knowing that I will ultimately have the ostomy reversed gave me hope and something to look forward to throughout my rehabilitation.

Permanent Ostomies

A permanent ostomy involves removing a part of the digestive or urinary system that cannot be rejoined. This is often the case when major sections of the colon are removed owing to colorectal cancer, or when the bladder is removed due to bladder cancer. Permanent ostomies require patients to have an ostomy pouch for the rest of their lives.

- Purpose: To bypass or replace dysfunctional parts of the colon or bladder.
- Duration: Permanent.
- Common Conditions: Colorectal cancer, severe inflammatory bowel disease, and bladder cancer.

Preoperative Considerations

Preparing for ostomy surgery extends beyond the physical. There is a lot to consider in terms of your mental health, emotional preparedness, and practical plans. Here are some tips to help you be as prepared as possible on the day of surgery.

1. Mental and emotional preparation for surgery

It is totally natural to feel a variety of emotions before ostomy surgery, including worry, anxiety, grief, and even rage. I recall feeling as if I was losing a piece of myself, a version of myself that was about to alter forever. Mental and emotional preparation are essential for managing these emotions, and it is OK to seek assistance if you are suffering.

Here are some mental and emotional preparation strategies:

- ✓ Speak with a Professional: Counseling or therapy may help you process your feelings about this life-changing procedure. Talking to a mental health expert who has worked with ostomy patients might help you build coping techniques.
- ✓ Join a Support Group: Connecting with others who have had ostomy surgery is really beneficial. Online forums, social media groups, and local ostomy support groups may provide encouragement, advice, and firsthand experiences.
- ✓ Research and educate yourself: Knowledge is power. Understanding the operation, rehabilitation, and what living with an ostomy entails may help to alleviate anxiety. Books, leaflets, and resources from your surgeon or ostomy nurse may assist to reduce your fears.
- ✓ Embrace Your Support Network: Rely on family, friends, and caretakers. Having someone to speak to, who can accompany you to appointments and provide emotional support, can make a significant difference.

2. Dietary Planning and Recommendations

In the weeks before surgery, your surgeon may provide dietary suggestions to prepare your digestive system for the operation. This usually includes:

- Low-Residue Diet: Prior to surgery, your doctor may suggest a low-fiber, low-residue diet to limit the quantity of waste traveling through your gut. This may make the procedure simpler and less complicated.

- Hydration: It's critical to remain hydrated in the days preceding up to surgery, especially if you've been having digestive troubles or diarrhea.
- Bowel Preparation: Depending on the kind of ostomy, your surgeon may require a bowel prep to empty up your intestines before the procedure. This generally entails drinking a specific solution to cleanse the intestines, comparable to preparing for a colonoscopy.

Your surgeon will offer precise advice, but it is critical to follow them closely to ensure that the treatment goes as well as possible.

3. What to bring to the hospital

Packing for a hospital stay may be stressful, but planning ahead of time can help alleviate tension. Here are some basics you should consider taking with you:

- Comfortable, Loose Clothing: Following surgery, you'll want garments that are simple to put on and soft on your abdomen. Loose pajamas, button-down shirts, and elastic-waist trousers are perfect.
- Personal amenities: Bring travel-sized amenities, such as a toothbrush, toothpaste, face wipes, and deodorant, to make yourself more comfortable.
- Ostomy Supplies (If provided): While some hospitals will give ostomy supplies, it's a good idea to bring any you've previously gotten, just in case. Being familiar with your own materials might provide comfort.
- Notebook or Journal: You'll learn a lot from nurses and physicians throughout your hospital stay. A notebook may help you write down vital data, queries, and directions for ostomy care.
- Entertainment: Recovery may be slow, so bring novels, a tablet, headphones, or your favorite music to pass the time.
- Supportive Items: Anything that gives comfort, such as a picture of a loved one, a favorite blanket, or a pillow, will help make your stay less stressful.

Postoperative Care in the Hospital

Waking up after ostomy surgery may be a difficult experience, both physically and emotionally. The time spent in the hospital after surgery is critical for recovering, learning how to care for your new stoma, and acquiring the confidence you'll need to live life with an ostomy.

Post-Surgical Experience: The First 24 Hours

It is normal to feel bewildered when you initially wake up after surgery. The bright lights, antiseptic odor of the hospital, and beeping devices might make it difficult to digest information. You may still feel foggy from the anesthetic, and you will most likely have tubes and monitors linked to you to watch your vital signs and assist with your recuperation.

I distinctly recall the moment I awoke. The first thing I felt was an odd pulling on my abdomen—not painful, just unusual. I reached down and touched the ostomy pouch, which had an unusual feel. It was genuine. I had read everything about it and mentally prepared myself, but nothing prepared me for the moment I touched it. My hand froze, and for a brief moment, I felt terror. What did I do? How was I expected to live with this? But then I took a breath, and reality sank in. I was not alone. In the distance, I could hear my nurse comforting me that I had done well and that we would proceed gradually. That confidence made all the difference in those early stages.

In the first few hours following surgery, you are likely to experience:

- Drowsiness and confusion: This is a frequent side effect of anesthesia, and your mind may take many hours to clear.
- Pain and discomfort: You will be given pain medicine, either via an IV or a patient-controlled analgesia (PCA) pump, which enables you to administer the drug yourself (within certain restrictions).
- Stoma Awareness: You will likely be introduced to your stoma for the first time. Do not be frightened if it seems bloated or blazing red; this is normal. Your stoma will shrink and heal with time.
- Monitors and drains: You may have drainage tubes installed to avoid fluid accumulation and promote recovery. You'll also have an ostomy bag linked to your stoma to collect waste.

The first 24 hours are important for your body to start mending. You will be continuously followed by medical professionals, and although you may feel vulnerable, each second is a step closer to recovery.

Manage Pain, Fatigue, and Side Effects

1. Pain management

Pain after surgery is unavoidable, but controlling it efficiently is critical for recovery. Pain might result from the incision, manipulation of your internal organs, or the existence of a stoma.

Following surgery, you may get intravenous (IV) pain medication. If you use a PCA pump, you may deliver the medicine whenever you need it.
- Oral pain medication: As your recovery develops, your doctor may switch you to oral pain medications.

It is critical to discuss freely with your healthcare provider about your pain level. Don't attempt "toughing it out." Effective pain treatment will allow you to move about sooner, which is critical for avoiding problems such as blood clots or pneumonia. Early movement is also important for your overall recovery.

I had heard stories of post-surgery discomfort and felt I could mentally prepare, but the reality was more painful than I anticipated. It wasn't continuous, but it came in waves, and it sometimes surprised me when I went in the incorrect direction. I was reluctant to ask for extra pain medicine because I thought it would be a display of weakness. But then, my nurse, who had been at my side since I awoke, saw my anguish and reminded me that pain management is about healing, not courage. When I let go of the notion that I had to be strong in the face of suffering, I was able to relax and concentrate on healing.

2. Fatigue

Fatigue after surgery might be severe. Your body is using a lot of energy to mend itself, and even basic acts like getting up in bed or taking a few steps may seem laborious. You'll probably require a lot of rest in the days after surgery.

To manage weariness, listen to your body. Rest as much as possible, but also listen to your healthcare staff when they advise you to exercise.
- Short walks: With help, move around your hospital room or down the corridor. Walking prevents issues such as blood clots and allows your digestive system to resume normal function.
- Remain hydrated: Dehydration may increase tiredness. Drink water or electrolyte-rich beverages as prescribed by your medical staff.

3. Managing Side Effects

Following ostomy surgery, adverse symptoms are prevalent. These may include:

- Nausea is a common adverse effect of anesthesia. Medications might be given to aid with nausea. You'll most likely be on a liquid diet until your digestive system recovers.
- Gas and bloating: It is common to have gas or bloating as your digestive system adapts to the changes. Over time, your body will adjust to its new normal.
- Changes in bowel movements: If you have undergone a colostomy or ileostomy, it may take a few days for your intestine to resume normal function. When it happens, the first emission might be liquid or gas.

Understanding the Role of the Stoma Nurse or Wound, Ostomy, and Continence (WOC) Nurse

Your stoma nurse or WOC (Wound, Ostomy, and Continence) nurse is an invaluable resource throughout your hospital stay. These professional nurses are trained to care for ostomy patients and teach them how to maintain their stoma and pouch system. They will play an important role in your recovery, teaching you how to care for your ostomy after you leave the hospital.

A stoma nurse teaches patients how to empty and replace their ostomy pouch, clean their stoma, and identify infection or problems. They will also explain what typical output looks like for your specific kind of ostomy.

- Emotional Support: Ostomy surgery may have a substantial emotional effect. Your stoma nurse will provide comfort and assistance as you adapt to this new part of your body. They've seen it all before and can address any questions or concerns without passing judgment.
- Troubleshooting: If you have any problems with your stoma, such as leakage, skin irritation, or difficulties with the pouch system, your stoma nurse will assist you in finding solutions.

My WOC nurse, Lisandra, was a lifesaver. Her calm, informed presence made a significant impact in my room from the time she entered. The first time she taught me how to change my bag, I was too afraid to touch it. What if I did anything wrong? What happens if I harm myself? But Lisandra had a knack of breaking things down into little, manageable chunks. She would add, "It's just like learning how to tie your shoes." It's awkward at first, but you'll get used to it." And she was correct. By the conclusion of my hospital stay, I wasn't an expert, but I knew enough to be confident. Lisandra's kindness, support, and competence transformed what seemed overwhelming into something I could manage.

Why a Stoma Nurse is Important

The stoma nurse plays an important role in the transition from hospital to home care. Without their direction, care with an ostomy might be daunting. They assist to normalize the procedure by reminding you that, with time and experience, maintaining your ostomy will become second nature.

Key takeaways

- Immediate Post-Surgery Experience: You should expect some disorientation, grogginess, and pain in the first 24 hours following surgery, but this is typical. Nurses and physicians will be available to assist you with pain management and answering any questions you may have.
- Pain and Fatigue Management: Do not be afraid to seek pain relief and listen to your body when it comes to resting. Small activities, like walking, are necessary for healing, but do it slowly.

- Stoma Nurse Support: The job of the stoma nurse is critical. They will educate you all you need to know about caring for your stoma and provide emotional support while you adapt.

It is common to feel overwhelmed by all of the new information in the days after your operation. But remember, you're not alone. You will make it through this with the help of your medical team, loved ones, and your own strength.

Part 2: The Emotional Experience

Ostomy surgery is more than simply a physical treatment; it also signals the start of a significant emotional journey. Coming to grips with a new reality is seldom simple. The transition to living with a stoma often elicits a variety of emotions, from denial and rage to acceptance. For many people, emotional scars may be just as severe as physical ones. But it is also an experience of resilience, bravery, and self-discovery.

Emotional Adjustment Stages: Coping with a New Reality

Following ostomy surgery, you may go through numerous phases of emotional adjustment. It is important to know that these emotions are legitimate, and many people who have this operation have similar experiences. The progression through these phases is not linear; some individuals may go through them numerous times, while others may bypass them entirely.

1. Denial

Denial is often the first response people have when they learn they require ostomy surgery or wake up with a stoma. It's difficult to realize that your body has transformed so dramatically. You may convince yourself that it is just temporary, or you may find it difficult to accept the necessity for an ostomy.

When the doctor informed me that I would require an ostomy, I nodded as if I understood. But the fact is that I didn't. I couldn't handle it. I left the office thinking they'd made a mistake, and that there could be another alternative they hadn't considered. For the first two weeks, I was unable to look at my stoma. I concealed it with additional garments, avoided mirrors, and pretended it didn't exist. However, the more I disregarded it, the more alienated I felt. I turned away individuals who wanted to assist me because I didn't want to admit what had occurred. It took some time for me to understand that suppressing my reality was not going to make things easier.

How to Deal with Denial

- Recognize your emotions: It is OK to express that you are struggling to embrace your new situation. This is a significant life adjustment that will take time to adjust to.
- Speak to others: Share your emotions with others who care about you, whether it's a loved one or a counselor. Denial flourishes in quiet, but when you open up, it loses its grasp.

2. Anger

As the reality of living with an ostomy becomes more apparent, anger is a normal reaction. You may be furious with your body for "betraying" you, the ailment or condition that brought you to this point, or even the medical personnel for conducting the operation despite the fact that it was required.

I'll be honest: I was furious after my operation. Really furious. It was unjust that I had to deal with this. So, why me? So, why now? I'd done everything "right." I exercised and ate well, yet none of it prevented me from ending up here. There were days when I snapped at my family for no apparent reason. I despised their capacity to live regular lives while mine had been permanently altered. It wasn't only the physical suffering; it was also the emotional toll, which seemed impossible to endure. I was furious with everyone and everything, but most of all, I was upset at myself for feeling like this.

Managing Anger

- Allow yourself to experience it: Don't hide your rage. It's an understandable and reasonable reaction to a major life shift.

- Journaling or consulting with a therapist might help you process your emotions in a healthy manner.
- Transform it into something positive: After you've vented your anger, attempt to channel it into something beneficial. Physical exercise, whether it's a brief stroll or a yoga session, may help reduce some of the stress associated with rage.

3. Acceptance

Acceptance does not imply liking or being satisfied with your ostomy. It simply implies that you have accepted that this is your new normal and are ready to find a way to go on. This stage might provide a feeling of calm as you begin to regain your life and adjust to the changes.

It didn't happen quickly, but I ultimately learned to embrace my ostomy. I recall looking in the mirror and not being repulsed or unhappy. Instead, I felt proud. I was proud of what my body had gone through, as well as the fortitude it required to get to the other side. Acceptance for me was not about seeing the ostomy as a positive—it was about coming to terms with the reality that it saved my life. I began to consider all I could accomplish now that I was well again. I felt myself slowly coming back to life.

- Celebrate tiny victories: Recognize your progress, whether it's learning to change your pouch on your own or venturing out in public for the first time after surgery.
- Network with others: Find ostomy sufferers' support organizations or internet communities. Hearing their tales of perseverance and courage might make you feel less alone and inspire your own path to acceptance.

Dealing With Loss or Body Image Changes

Ostomy surgery may cause physical changes that have a significant impact on how you see yourself. It is normal to feel a sense of loss—loss of your pre-surgery physique, independence, or even control over your life. These emotions are often linked to shifts in body image. Following surgery, you may feel detached from your body or struggle to accept its new shape.

1. Dealing with Loss

It is acceptable to lament the loss of your body as it was before surgery. You may feel as if your body has altered so much that it is unrecognizable. For some people, an ostomy may serve as a visual reminder of sickness or trauma, complicating the mental recovery process.

I wept for the life I believed I had lost. In the days and weeks after my surgery, I couldn't help but reflect on all the things I had taken for granted, such as being able to wear my favorite clothing without thinking about how my pouch would appear beneath. I felt like a piece of me had been ripped away, and I wasn't sure whether I'd ever get it back. But one day, a friend came by and gave me a gift: a new dress that was beautiful, comfortable, and suited my ostomy. She reminded me that, although I had lost a part of me, I had gained something else—a shot at life. Slowly, I began to concentrate on what I had gained rather than what I had lost.

- Recognize your grief: It is OK to grieve the loss of your pre-surgery physique or lifestyle. Allow yourself to be sad and take time to recover emotionally.
- Focus on what you've learned**: While the surgery may have altered your physical appearance, it most likely saved your life or enhanced your quality of life. Shifting your focus from loss to survival might help alleviate the emotional weight.

2. Addressing Changes in Body Image

The alterations to your body after surgery might have a significant influence on how you see yourself. Suddenly, you may feel strange, self-conscious, or even embarrassed of your looks. Ostomy patients often battle with body image issues, but there are methods to restore confidence and learn to love their bodies again.

I'm not going to lie—I sobbed the first time I saw my stoma. It wasn't what I anticipated, and I couldn't see how I'd ever feel at ease in my flesh again. But, over time, something extraordinary occurred. I recognized that the stoma, as alien and foreign as it seemed, represented my power. It embodied all I had gone through and overcome. Instead of concealing it, I began embracing it. I discovered things that made me feel attractive and confident, and I even began to open up about my experiences. When I stopped allowing my ostomy to determine my value, I started reclaiming my body image.

- Dress comfortably and confidently. Many firms now provide fashionable apparel alternatives exclusively for ostomy sufferers.
- Practice self-compassion: Remember that your body has gone through a lot, and it deserves care and patience while it recovers. Treat your body with dignity and care
- Celebrate your resilience: Your physique reflects your strength and capacity to conquer obstacles. Accept the scars and changes as part of your own experience.

Moving Forward with Emotional Healing

The emotional experience after ostomy surgery is not easy, but it is one of development, strength, and rediscovery. It's natural to experience a variety of emotions, including denial, rage, despair, and even relief. Each emotion is a normal part of the healing process, and you will eventually come to embrace yourself. It's also vital to realize that you don't have to face this alone. Lean on your support system, which may include friends, family, healthcare professionals, or other ostomy patients.

Your emotional well-being is as crucial as your physical healing. As you embark on this new chapter in your life, be nice to yourself and believe that emotional healing will occur with time and patience.

Restoring Confidence and Self-Worth

Coming to grips with life after ostomy surgery is learning to recover your self-esteem and confidence. This is not something that occurs suddenly, but rather as a slow process of rediscovering. It's normal to believe that your body has betrayed you or that you've lost a piece of your identity. The next step is to learn to recover your identity and accept the power you've earned along the way.

1. Redefine Your Self-Worth

Many individuals associate confidence with body image, health, and physical aptitude. After ostomy surgery, it's tempting to believe that your value has lessened since your body looks or operates differently than before. However, genuine self-worth comes from inside, and acknowledging this may be quite motivating.

I recall looking in the mirror and realizing I was focused on the wrong things. I was so focused on what I'd lost that I entirely overlooked what I'd gained. My body had been through a battle, yet here I was—alive and going ahead. That moment signaled a change in how I saw myself. Instead of seeing my ostomy as a fault or something that made me inferior, I came to see it as a symbol of my strength. My value stemmed from my capacity to endure and grow in the face of adversity, not from possessing a "perfect" physique.

- Focus on your strengths: Your worth is not dependent on your physical attractiveness. Take time to appreciate the inner traits that define you—kindness, intellect, humor, and resilience.
- Get involved in things that make you feel accomplished: Whether it's a pastime, a career, or volunteering, find something that makes you feel helpful and satisfied.
- Celebrate Your Survival: Living with an ostomy does not imply weakness; rather, it demonstrates that you have overcome hardship. Take pride in your path.

2. Reclaim Your Life

An ostomy may alter the way you live, but it does not have to prevent you from living completely. The goal is to learn to adapt and make modifications as needed, without letting your ostomy define or constrain you. Whether it's going back to work, interacting with friends, or doing your favorite hobbies, regaining your life is an important aspect of the emotional healing process.

One of my greatest concerns after the operation was that I would never be able to do the activities I enjoyed again. I was a very active person who enjoyed hiking and traveling, and the prospect of doing so with an ostomy was daunting. However, after a few months, I decided to take a risk. I began modestly, taking little walks around the neighborhood. Then one day, I went hiking with a good buddy. We packed everything I needed for my ostomy, and I was amazed by how natural it felt. It was empowering to learn that, although I needed to prepare more, I could still participate in things that made me feel alive. That was the day I stopped allowing my ostomy to hold me back.

- Take one step at a time. Begin with tiny objectives and work your way back to things you like.
- Do not be scared to ask for assistance: Whether you're discussing modifications with your healthcare team or seeking support from friends and family, remember that you don't have to go through this alone.
- Celebrate each victory: Every step forward, no matter how tiny, is an accomplishment worth celebrating.

Developing Emotional Resilience

The emotional path after ostomy surgery is full of ups and downs. While the first few months might be difficult, many individuals come away with a newfound feeling of emotional resiliency. Developing emotional resilience entails learning to deal with setbacks and emerge stronger on the other side.

I used to believe that emotional resilience was something you had or did not have. But following my operation, I discovered that resilience is something you can develop one day at a time. At first, everything was overpowering, and I wondered how I'd ever feel normal again. But as the days passed, I discovered modest methods to retake control of my life. I began journaling to help me process my feelings. I also joined an online support group to connect with people going through similar situations. Things that looked overwhelming at first were more doable as time passed. I was not simply surviving; I was flourishing.

To build emotional resilience, practice mindfulness and self-care via activities such as meditation, yoga, or writing.

- Connect with others: Attending support groups, whether in person or online, may give you a feeling of belonging and remind you that you are not alone on your path.
- Focus on what you control: There may be parts of your ostomy that you cannot change, but there are other areas of your life that you can.

Concentrate on those areas and make positive changes to increase your well-being.

This experience might be challenging, but it will expose your inner power and tenacity. Throughout the highs and lows, you will uncover new elements of yourself that you were previously unaware of. Accepting your body, regaining your self-esteem, and recovering the things you like are all steps toward recovery. Finally, you'll realize that your ostomy, however tough, is just one aspect of the lovely, complicated person you are.

Coping Strategies for Emotional Wellbeing

Living with an ostomy may cause a flood of emotions. From anguish over a loss of normality to concern about how life will unfold in the future, the emotional journey may often seem as important as the physical one. Coping with these emotional ups and downs is essential for not just existing but flourishing with your ostomy.

Journalizing and Expressing Feelings

Journaling is one of the easiest and most effective methods to process emotions. Writing helps us to express sentiments that may otherwise stay suppressed. Many people who have had ostomy surgery find that writing down their thoughts helps them make sense of their emotional journey.

When you're overwhelmed, confused, or experiencing a deluge of emotions, writing allows you to calm down and reflect. It's a private, personal outlet that may bring significant relief by enabling you to measure your progress, celebrate your achievements, and get a deeper understanding of the problems.

I began writing a few weeks following my operation, more out of desperation than anything. I was weary of carrying around so many emotions—anger, anxiety, and frustration—with no meaningful release. Writing became my means of communicating with myself without judgment. One night, when I was particularly down, I penned a letter to my pre-surgery self. It was a combination of mourning and encouragement, letting go of what I'd lost but simultaneously acknowledging how far I'd come. That letter proved to be a turning moment for me. It helped me recognize that, although my life had altered, it was not finished. *I could still write the following chapter.

- Begin with a daily reflection: Make writing a daily habit, whether it's a single line or a complete page. Consider how you're feeling emotionally and physically. Over time, you'll see trends and progress.
- Don't censor yourself. Your diary is a judgment-free zone. Write everything that comes to mind, no matter how raw or unedited.
- Explore several formats: If words don't come freely, try alternative forms of communication, such as doodling, poetry, or lists. The idea is to express your emotions, not to compose a polished essay.

Mindfulness Practices and Relaxation Techniques

When life seems stressful, mindfulness may provide much-needed relief. Mindfulness entails being completely present in the moment, without judgment. For someone adapting to life with an ostomy, mindfulness may help navigate the emotional ups and downs by focusing on the now rather than worrying about the future or regretting the past.

It is not necessary to follow a complex regimen to practice mindfulness. Simple approaches such as concentrating on your breath, participating in guided meditation, or simply taking a mindful stroll may have a major impact on your mental well-being. Deep breathing and progressive muscle relaxation are two relaxation strategies that may assist with stress and anxiety reduction.

One day, when I was feeling especially nervous about my new life, a buddy advised me to try mindfulness meditation. I was hesitant at first—I didn't see how sitting motionless would help me absorb the weight of my emotions. But I gave it a try. I recall sitting on my sofa, eyes closed, and concentrating exclusively on my breathing. Inhale, exhale. My mind's chatter gradually became quieter. Worries about how people might judge me, and if I'd ever feel 'normal' again, began to vanish. For a few seconds, I was just there, and it seemed as if a weight had been lifted. Since then, mindfulness has been a part of my daily routine, providing me with a means to center myself when life becomes chaotic.*

- Focus on deep breathing for five minutes. Inhale for four counts, hold for four, and then exhale for four. This little practice may provide immediate relaxation.

- Lie down or sit comfortably and focus on each area of your body, beginning with your toes and progressing to your head. Notice any tightness and intentionally release it as you travel through each location.
- Select anything in your surroundings—a flower, a tree, or even your cup of tea. Observe it without judgment, seeing its nuances and enjoying it for what it is.

The Importance of Therapy or Counseling

While personal coping strategies such as journaling and mindfulness may be quite effective, there are instances when professional assistance is required. Therapy or counseling may offer a structured setting for working with the complicated emotions that often develop after ostomy surgery. This might include emotions of loss, anger, or solitude, which are difficult to handle on their own.

A therapist or counselor, especially one with expertise in chronic disease or post-surgical care, may help you develop coping techniques and validate your emotions. Group therapy or support groups may also help you connect with people who understand what you're going through.

- Safe place for processing emotions: Therapy offers a judgment-free atmosphere to explore emotions without burdening loved ones.
- Learning coping strategies: A professional may teach you new techniques for dealing with ostomy-related stress, anxiety, or despair.
- Creating a Support Network: Connecting with people who understand your experience, whether via individual or group therapy, may help you feel less alone.

Different types of treatment include cognitive-behavioral therapy (CBT). CBT assists people in changing negative thought habits and replacing them with more constructive ways of thinking.

- Group Therapy: In a group environment, you may discuss your experiences with others who have had similar surgery, creating a feeling of community.

- Online Support Groups: If visiting therapy in person seems overwhelming, there are various online forums where individuals may discuss their experiences and provide support.

Remember that your feelings are legitimate. It's acceptable to feel sad, angry, or overwhelmed sometimes. What counts most is how you deal with those sensations and whether you seek the assistance and support you need.

Talking with Family and Friends

For many individuals who have had ostomy surgery, one of the most difficult aspects of the emotional journey is explaining it to their loved ones. How do you address the reality that you now have a stoma? How will they respond? What if they don't understand, or worse, have a negative reaction?

Explaining Your Stoma to Loved Ones

Explaining an ostomy to relatives and friends might be scary. The issue is to explain a complicated medical condition without overwhelming your loved ones or causing agony on either side. However, honesty is essential here. Being open and honest with people closest to you may provide the groundwork for mutual understanding and support.

When you decide to explain your stoma, consider this easy, uncomplicated approach:

1. Use intelligible language: Begin with basic facts. "I underwent surgery that resulted in a stoma, a tiny incision in my belly through which my body may now transfer waste. This was important to enhance my health because... (Enter the reason for your operation, such as cancer, Crohn's disease, or injuries)."
2. Prepare for inquiries: It is typical for loved ones to have questions about ostomies, particularly if they are unfamiliar with them. You may hear "What does it look like?" or "How does it work?" Be prepared to answer their questions patiently and explain them as much as you feel comfortable.
3. Highlight your needs: It is critical to clarify how they can help you, whether it is by providing emotional support or recognizing that you may need extra time for self-care, particularly throughout the healing process.

I recall the day I informed my best buddy about my stoma. I was scared, afraid she wouldn't know how to respond. I said, 'I need to tell you something crucial regarding my health.' She stared at me with worry, and the words stuck in my throat. However, when I told that I now had a stoma, she just nodded and said, 'What can I do to help?' It was hardly the reaction I had dreaded. It was a relief, and at that moment, I knew how important open communication is. By being open, I gained an ally rather than losing a friend.

How to Deal with Reactions and Stigma

Everyone handles medical conditions differently. Some of your loved ones may react quickly with sympathy and interest. Others may be uneasy, unsure how to respond or what to say. Unfortunately, others may react with ignorance or even judgment, motivated by cultural stigma or misunderstanding of ostomies.

It's crucial to realize that their emotions do not represent your value or identity. You have no control over how people react, but you can manage and negotiate these interactions.

`Common Reactions:`

- Supportive and empathetic: These individuals listen without judgment, ask insightful questions, and provide unconditional support. These individuals are your emotional lifelines.
- Uncomfortable or unsure: Some loved ones may feel uncomfortable or uneasy at first, sometimes because of a lack of understanding regarding ostomies. These people often want further schooling to feel comfortable, and they are eager to study more once the topic is normalized.
- Stigma or judgment: Unfortunately, some people may respond out of ignorance or discomfort, displaying stigma against the concept of a stoma. They could comment, "That must be so embarrassing" or, "How do you deal with that?" While these statements might be hurtful, they are often the result of a misunderstanding.

I recall informing a family member, who was instantly appalled. Her reply was the very last thing I needed. 'Isn't that gross?' she said. I anticipated inquiries, but not judgment. It was painful, and for a long time I wondered whether I should have said anything at all. But then I understood her response was not about me, but about her discomfort. I decided to educate her, telling her more about my experiences. To my astonishment, she became softer with time. She even apologized afterward, confessing that she didn't know much about ostomies and had responded harshly due to ignorance. This showed me that sometimes individuals just need time and knowledge to catch up.

- Remember your value. Your stoma does not define you, and it is not your responsibility to bear the incapacity of others to realize this.
- Set limits: If someone constantly makes insensitive or cruel statements, it is OK to establish hard boundaries. Inform them that their remarks have an impact on you and that their responses are unacceptable.
- Seek help elsewhere: If a specific loved one is unable to give the necessary assistance, look for others who can. This might include other family members, friends, or support groups.

Educate Those around You

Educating your family and friends about your stoma is about more than simply refuting myths; it's about fostering an atmosphere of understanding and acceptance. When others understand your medical condition and the reasons behind it, they might be more supportive.

Education also minimizes the mystery and stigma associated with medical devices such as stomas. Many people are unfamiliar with ostomies and may have misunderstandings, such as believing they are unsanitary or that persons with ostomies cannot live regular lives. The more knowledgeable your loved ones are, the more prepared they will be to be by your side and support you.

How to Educate Your Loved Ones:

1. Provide simple resources: People may feel too ashamed to ask straightforward inquiries. Offering basic brochures or online resources may provide customers with the necessary knowledge without putting you under pressure to answer every inquiry.

2. Open dialogue: Encourage open interactions in which family members feel comfortable expressing questions. Tell them it's good to be interested, and that you admire their want to learn.
3. Relate your experiences: Don't be hesitant to relate your own path, even the difficult moments. Being vulnerable allows people to better appreciate the emotional and physical reality of living with a stoma.

When I mentioned my stoma to my family, I wasn't sure how detailed I wanted to go. However, I discovered that the more I revealed, the more comfortable they were. My sister was extremely inquisitive, so I showed her one of the instructional movies I received following surgery. She asked a lot of questions, and I liked her desire to understand what I was going through. Over time, I observed a change. What began as curiosity soon evolved into empathy, and I could feel her support getting stronger. My family became my strongest supporters once I took the effort to educate them.

Addressing Common Myths about Ostomies:

- Myth: Ostomies are unsanitary.
    - Reality: A stoma and its surrounding region are supposed to be as clean as possible. People with ostomies take care of their stomachs and use specialist products to keep them clean and controlled.

Most persons with ostomies may continue their usual activities, including employment, exercise, and travel. With time, many individuals discover that they can accomplish what they used to do and more.

- Myth: Stomas are unusual and aberrant.
    - Reality: Ostomies are more frequent than most people realize. Thousands of people throughout the globe have ostomies owing to illnesses such as Crohn's disease, cancer, and injuries. There's nothing to be embarrassed of.

Explaining your ostomy to family and friends may be difficult, but it is a necessary step toward developing a solid support network. When your loved ones understand your situation, they can provide the understanding and care you need throughout your rehabilitation and beyond.

Not everyone will respond in the manner you expect, but those who genuinely care will listen, ask intelligent questions, and show up for you in significant ways. And by educating others around you, you are helping to break the stigma associated with ostomies, paving the path for those who may face the same road in the future.

Remember, you're not simply discussing a medical problem; you're also promoting connection and understanding. By telling your experience with honesty and bravery, you make room for people who love you to stand by your side.

Part 3: Understanding your Stoma

Living with a stoma may be a difficult adjustment, but the more you understand it, the more power you have over your care and well-being.

Anatomy of the Stoma: What it is and how it works

When a stoma develops, a section of the intestine or urinary system is brought through the abdominal wall. This little incision, often reddish or pink in color, is then secured to the skin. A stoma bag, sometimes known as an ostomy equipment, is fitted to the outside to collect waste. It is critical to remember that the stoma itself has no nerve endings, hence there is no feeling when it is touched.

How Stomas Work:

A stoma creates a new pathway for body waste to leave. Because the muscles in the digestive or urinary systems that govern elimination are bypassed, waste is expelled involuntarily. There are no sphincters or valves to restrict feces or urine passing through the stoma, therefore output is continuous, requiring the adoption of a pouching device to collect waste. The stoma lets waste exit the body effectively, protecting it from the negative consequences of accumulating waste.

When I first awoke after surgery and saw my stoma, I was overcome with emotion." I was relieved that the operation was successful, but I was also overwhelmed by this new portion of my body. At first, I couldn't even look at it, much alone grasp how it operated. However, when I learned more about its function, I concluded that my stoma was nothing to be afraid of. It really saved my life. And, although it took some time to get accustomed to seeing it, I now see it as a symbol of survival and tenacity.*

End or Loop Stomas

Stomas are not all constructed the same way, and knowing the distinctions between an end stoma and a loop stoma will help you understand why your stoma looks and works as it does.

End Stoma

End stomas are the most frequent form of stoma. It is formed when one end of the intestine is brought through the abdominal wall while the remainder of the intestine is removed or rendered inactive inside the body. This kind of stoma is often used for permanent ostomies, such as when the rectum or bladder are no longer functioning or have been removed owing to illness. The stoma has just one entrance through which all waste travels.

Loop Stoma

A loop stoma is often formed as a temporary remedy, particularly when the surgeon intends to reattach the intestines at a later date. In a loop stoma, a loop of the intestine is introduced through the abdominal wall and partly opened, resulting in two stoma openings: one for waste escape and another for connecting to the remainder of the bowel and enabling it to rest. As a result, loop stomas might be bigger and more difficult to maintain than end stomas.

While in recuperation, I discovered that my stoma was a loop ileostomy. This signified that the doctors intended to undo it once my intestines recovered. It gave me hope, knowing that my circumstance was just transitory, but it also presented obstacles. Because my stoma had two openings, regulating the outflow seemed harder, and I struggled at first. But my stoma nurse was fantastic, teaching me how to care for it and adapt to its specific requirements.

Prolapsed and Retracted Stomas

Complications might emerge that impact how a stoma appears and functions. Prolapsed and retracted stomata are two prevalent conditions. While these illnesses may seem serious, they are usually treatable with the proper treatment and medical assistance.

Collapsed Stoma

A prolapsed stoma occurs when the intestine extends farther out of the belly than it should, causing the stoma to seem elongated or protruding more than usual. Coughing or straining might cause increased abdominal pressure. While a prolapsed stoma may seem alarming, it is generally treatable without surgery. In rare situations, the stoma may retract on its own, but a medical assessment is required to rule out any issues like blockages or impaired blood flow.

Retraction

A retracted stoma occurs when the stoma pushes inward, bringing it flush with or under the skin's surface. This may be troublesome since it makes it more difficult to firmly connect an ostomy pouch and raises the possibility of leakage or skin irritation. A retracted stoma may be caused by weight fluctuations, scar tissue, or specific postures that alter the location of the abdominal muscles. In some circumstances, adjusting the ostomy equipment might assist, while others may need surgical intervention.

One of the worst moments for me following surgery was discovering that my stoma had prolapsed. It looked so different from before, and I was terrified. I recall wondering, "Is this normal?" Is there anything wrong? Fortunately, my stoma nurse told me that prolapsed stomas are a somewhat frequent problem and that it was not an emergency. She showed me how to modify my pouching system to fit the alteration, and after a few weeks, it began retracting on its own. It was a reminder that the stoma, like the rest of my body, might alter over time, which is OK.

Normal Appearance versus When to Seek Help

One of the most significant components of living with a stoma is getting to know what it should look like on a regular basis so you can spot problems. Regular stoma monitoring will help you identify any concerns early on, enabling you to seek urgent medical attention.

How a Healthy Stoma Looks

A stoma is a surgically formed orifice that, although strange at first, seems normal and healthy as you get used to it. Knowing what your stoma should look like can help you be aware of any changes.

1. Color: A healthy stoma is often pinkish-red or deep red, similar to the interior of the mouth. Your stoma's bright, vascular look is due to the fact that it is constructed from a section of the intestine with a good blood supply. It's quite normal for the stoma to seem wet since it secretes mucus to aid with waste disposal. The color should be stable throughout time.

2. Shape: The size and shape of a stoma varies based on its location and operation type. The majority of stomas are round or oval in shape, and although some protrude slightly from the belly, others are flush with the skin.
- End stomas are normally circular, while loop stomas might be more oval or have two separate openings. As the edema following surgery subsides, your stoma may decrease somewhat, but the overall form will remain the same.

3. Stoma size varies based on parameters such as body type, operation kind, and intestinal location. Stomas normally measure 25 to 35 millimeters in diameter, they might be bigger or smaller depending on your specific instance. Your stoma may be somewhat enlarged in the weeks after surgery, but this should subside over time to a more consistent size.

4. Texture: A healthy stoma is soft and wet. You may detect a small gloss on its surface as a result of the mucus it produces naturally. The stoma will have no nerve endings, thus touching or cleaning around it will not cause discomfort. This is crucial to remember, particularly when searching for abnormalities: you can inspect your stoma without causing pain.

5. Bleeding: It's common for a stoma to bleed somewhat when touched or cleaned. This is due to the high concentration of blood vessels on the surface, which might result in minor bleeding, particularly during pouch changes or if you accidently touch it. However, this bleeding should be modest and should subside rapidly

I was horrified when I first saw my stoma following surgery. It didn't look as I anticipated. It was brilliant red, wet, and felt strange to me. But, with time, I came to identify its natural look. I had frequent chats with my stoma nurse, who told me that it was healthy and that the brilliant red hue indicated strong blood flow. At first, I was scared when I noticed even the smallest amount of blood during pouch changes, but understanding that a little bleeding was typical set my mind at rest.

When to Seek Help: Signs of Potential Issues

While it is natural for your stoma to appear in a specific manner, it is also crucial to notice when anything is wrong. Catching possible concerns early may assist to avoid more significant difficulties. Here are several warning indicators that need quick treatment from your healthcare physician.

1. Excessive bleeding

Light bleeding when cleaning or replacing your appliance is typical; however, you should seek medical attention if you have continuous bleeding or observe blood in your stool or urine (depending on the kind of stoma). Excessive bleeding may indicate blood vessel damage around the stoma, an infection, or some underlying condition. If the bleeding does not stop within a few minutes, or if the blood is black or clotted, contact your doctor right once.

2. Color changes

A healthy stoma appears pink or crimson, suggesting adequate blood flow. If your stoma becomes purple, black, or dark blue, it might indicate that its blood supply is impaired. Such discoloration may be caused by stoma necrosis, which occurs when tissue starts to die owing to insufficient circulation. A pale stoma may indicate inadequate blood flow, but a deeper hue may indicate severe blockage or pressure. If you detect any changes in hue, get medical treatment right away.

3. Sudden Changes in Size and Shape

Your stoma's size may alter somewhat throughout the healing process after surgery, but any abrupt or severe changes are reason for worry. A swollen stoma that suddenly becomes bigger than usual may signal an obstruction, infection, or prolapse, in which the stoma pushes out of the body farther than normal. In contrast, if the stoma shrinks or retracts below the skin surface, it might raise the risk of skin irritation or infection. If you observe any abrupt size changes, contact your healthcare professional.

4. Prolapsed or retracted stoma

As discussed in Chapter 3, a prolapsed stoma occurs when the intestine protrudes more than usual, while a retracted stoma draws back into the abdomen. Both scenarios might make it harder to control your equipment and cause issues. If your stoma gets prolapsed or retracted, particularly if it occurs unexpectedly, you should have it checked by a medical practitioner. These disorders are sometimes treatable without surgery, but they must be evaluated to avoid future consequences.

5. Severe Pain around Stoma

While the stoma itself lacks nerve connections and should not cause pain, you may feel discomfort around the surrounding skin. However, if you have severe pain in the region, this might suggest an infection, abscess, or obstruction in your gut. Pain that lasts or worsens should be investigated by a doctor, particularly if it is accompanied by other symptoms like fever, edema, or redness around the stoma.

6. An unusual odor or discharge

While the waste that travels through your stoma will normally produce some odor, any foul or unusual odors emanating from the stoma or the surrounding skin may suggest an infection. Similarly, if you observe any pus-like discharge, especially near the base of the stoma, it's a symptom of infection or irritation that should be addressed right away. This may also be accompanied by redness or warmth at the stoma.

7. Skin irritation or breakdown

The skin surrounding your stoma, called as peristome skin, should be healthy and undamaged. It is normal for slight discomfort to occur on occasion, particularly if your appliance leaks, but persistent redness, sores, or skin breakdown around the stoma should be treated. Chronic inflammation might cause infections or more serious skin issues. If you're having trouble keeping the skin surrounding your stoma healthy, talk to your stoma nurse or healthcare provider about other pouching options or treatments.

Proactive Care: Steps to Follow

You may preserve your health and minimize issues by taking a proactive approach to stoma care and learning the usual vs abnormal indications. Here are a few actions you may take to keep your stoma healthy.

1. Inspect your stoma daily

Take a few minutes each day to examine your stoma and surrounding skin. Check for changes in color, size, and texture. Pay close attention to any unusual bleeding, scents, or discharges. This regular check will help you identify any problems before they become severe.

2. Stay hydrated

Staying hydrated is especially important for ileostomies since the stoma may cause you to lose more fluids than normal. Dehydration might impair your stomach's function and cause other health problems. Make sure you are drinking enough water throughout the day.

3. Eat a healthy diet

Adjusting your diet to accommodate your stoma is critical for maintaining good digestion and avoiding obstructions. Consult your doctor or nutritionist about which meals are best for your particular kind of ostomy. Certain meals may increase output or irritate your stoma, so experiment cautiously and track how your body responds to various foods.

4. Work with your Stoma Nurse

Your stoma nurse is a crucial member of your care team. Even after your initial recuperation, do not hesitate to contact them if you have any questions or concerns. If you're having issues with your stoma or appliances, your nurse can investigate the problem and propose remedies.

Stoma Care Basics

After surgery, you must care for your stoma on a regular basis. Creating a consistent regimen can help you maintain both physical comfort and cleanliness, avoiding difficulties like skin irritation or infection. For novices, learning how to correctly clean the stoma region and choose the appropriate solutions may seem intimidating, but with advice and experience, it becomes a manageable component of your self-care.

How to Clean Around Your Stoma

Cleaning the skin surrounding your stoma, known as the peristome region, is crucial to keeping it healthy. This fragile skin is susceptible to irritation from your stoma's output, but with careful care, it may be kept clean and healthy.

1. Gather your supplies

Before you begin cleaning your stoma, make sure you have all of the appropriate equipment around. This includes:

- Mild soap or cleaning wipes (make sure they are devoid of alcohol and smell).
- Warm Water
- Non-abrasive wipes or soft washcloths
- Stoma powder or barrier cream (if advised by your physician)
- Clean pouch and/or stoma appliance (if replacing during this procedure).
- Mirror (if necessary for increased visibility)

Having everything ready will allow you to work more efficiently and limit the amount of time your skin is exposed to air without protection.

2. Remove the old appliance carefully

If you're replacing your stoma pouch or appliance, begin by carefully removing the previous one. To prevent tugging at the skin, peel the glue away carefully, using your palm to support it. If the glue is really persistent, try an adhesive removal spray or wipe, but be sure to properly clean the area afterwards.

Dispose of the old pouch in a plastic bag or rubbish container, with any waste sealed to avoid smells.

3. Cleanse the skin

After removing the previous equipment, wipe the skin surrounding your stoma carefully with warm water and a soft cloth. Avoid using strong soaps or washing too hard since this region is delicate, and harsh products might cause inflammation. If you do use soap, be sure it is mild and has no alcohol, colors, or fragrances. Many individuals find it simpler to clean their stomachs when bathing since the water flows freely and gently rinses away waste.

Be thorough but delicate, and don't touch the stoma too much. The stoma lacks nerve endings, therefore touching it will not cause discomfort, but excessive handling may result in minor bleeding.

Pat the area dry

After washing, use a soft towel or cloth to gently dry the region surrounding the stoma. Before applying a new appliance, ensure that your skin is fully dry. Moisture may interfere with the adhesive, resulting in leaks or irritations.

5. Use a barrier product if necessary

If your skin is prone to inflammation, consider using a skin barrier or stoma powder. These products establish a protective covering on the skin, preventing injury from your stoma's output or the adhesive appliance.

For example, if your skin is raw or inflamed, stoma powder may help absorb moisture and soothe it. If your skin is deteriorating, a barrier film or protective wipes might provide further protection. Follow your healthcare provider's instructions for applying these items correctly.

6. Attach the New Appliance

Once your skin is clean and dry, apply your new stoma appliance. To avoid leaks, ensure that it fits securely around your stoma with no gaps between it and the adhesive. Depending on the kind of appliance, you may need to fasten it with an adhesive ring or belt to provide additional support.

Preventing and Treating Skin Irritation

The skin around your stoma is fragile and easily inflamed, particularly if it comes into touch with your stoma's discharge. Preventing and controlling irritation is essential for remaining comfortable and preventing illnesses. Here are some suggestions for keeping your peristome skin healthy.

1. Ensure the Proper Fit for Your Appliance

One of the most common causes of skin irritation is a poorly fitting stoma device. If the hole in the wafer or adhesive barrier is too big, the stoma's output may come into contact with your skin, causing discomfort or disintegration. If the appliance is too tiny, it may cut into and harm your stoma.

Your stoma is likely to vary size following surgery, especially in the first several weeks. Use a measurement guide to check your stoma's size on a regular basis, and ensure that your appliance fits securely. Your stoma nurse can teach you how to properly measure and choose the appropriate-sized device.

2. Use skin barriers

Barrier creams, sprays, or wipes help shield your skin from the outflow of your stoma. If your skin is easily irritated, using a barrier before attaching the appliance might help provide a protective layer between your skin and the adhesive. These creams are particularly beneficial if your skin is already showing indications of irritation, since they may reduce inflammation and prevent additional damage.

3. Avoid frequent appliance changes

Frequent removal and reapplication of your stoma device may cause skin wear and tear, especially if the adhesive is strong or you clean the region excessively. Try to strike a balance by changing your appliance on a regular enough basis to eliminate leaks but not so often that it irritates the skin. Most individuals find that they need to replace their appliance every 3 to 7 days. This varies depending on the kind of stoma and degree of activity.

4. Treat Skin Issues Early

If you observe any indications of skin irritation, such as redness, swelling, or itching, treat them as soon as possible to avoid further complications. A modest amount of redness may usually be alleviated by adjusting your appliance or using stoma powder, but more serious irritation may need medical treatment. Do not hesitate to contact your stoma nurse if your skin issues continue or worsen.

5. Avoid using lotions and oily products

Lotions, lotions, and greasy items might make it harder for your stoma device to adhere to your skin effectively, resulting in leaks. If your skin is dry, utilize items specialized for peristome skin care that will not interfere with the adhesive. Always check the labels to be sure they're safe to use with your equipment.

Selecting the Right Products for Your Needs

With so many stoma care items available, it's critical to choose the ones that best meet your specific requirements. Different stomachs and skin types need different items, and it may take some time to discover the appropriate mix of appliances and accessories that works for you. Here's how to browse your selections.

1. Types of Stoma Appliances

- One-Piece Systems: These appliances combine the adhesive wafer and pouch in a single item. They are simple to use and useful for those who value simplicity. One-piece systems are popular among individuals who desire fewer steps in their regimen, but they may be less adaptable for those who need to alter the wafer more regularly.
- Two-Piece Systems: These include a separate pouch and wafer, allowing you to replace the pouch without removing the adhesive from your skin. This is useful for folks who need to change their purse often or who want more flexibility. Two-piece systems may take longer to apply, but they may prevent skin irritation by decreasing the number of complete appliance changes.

2. Consider your activity level

If you are active or participate in strenuous activities, you will need a stoma appliance that offers additional protection. Look for extended-wear adhesives or convex wafers to provide a tighter fit and limit the possibility of leaks during movement. Some patients feel that wearing an ostomy belt adds additional support during exercise or sports.

3. Skin Type Matters

If you have sensitive skin, you should use products developed for mild care. Look for hypoallergenic adhesive barriers that are devoid of harmful substances. Some adhesives are designed to be softer on the skin, and adhesive removers may help make appliance changes less painful.

4. Use Accessory Products Wisely

Aside from the device itself, there are various accessories that may assist enhance your comfort and stoma care routine:

- Stoma Paste: This fills up crevices between your skin and the appliance, resulting in a better seal and less leaks.
- Barrier Rings: These soft, moldable rings provide a secure barrier between your stoma and appliance. They are useful for those with uneven skin contours or who want more leak protection.
- Deodorizing Drops: Place these in your bag to help neutralize scents and provide peace of mind in public settings.

Choosing the proper items was one of the toughest aspects of my stoma care experience. At first, I tried a variety of appliances, but none of them appeared to function completely for me. Some would irritate me, while others would not fit snugly enough. After a few months, with the aid of my stoma nurse, I discovered a two-piece device that provided both flexibility and security. Adding barrier rings to my regimen also helped reduce the leaks I'd been experiencing. It took some time, but the trial and error paid off—I'm finally comfortable with my stoma care regimen.

Part 4: Mastering Ostomy Care

Ostomy care is a continuous process that demands attention, patience, and adaptation. Understanding the various ostomy appliances available is an important part of caring for your stoma. Each system is meant to satisfy distinct demands, such as convenience, flexibility, or skin protection.

Ostomy Appliance

An ostomy appliance has two primary components: the pouch, which collects output from the stoma, and the adhesive barrier, which clings to your skin and forms a seal around the stoma. Appliances come in a variety of styles to suit individual tastes, activity levels, and skin types.

Understanding how these systems function and the alternatives available will let you choose a system that best meets your individual requirements, enabling you to live comfortably and confidently with your ostomy.

Understanding the many types of pouches

An ostomy pouch's principal role is to collect waste (usually feces or pee, depending on the kind of ostomy). While all pouches serve the same fundamental function, they exist in a variety of shapes and sizes, and the best one for you is determined by a number of criteria such as your stoma output, lifestyle, and personal preferences.

1-Piece Systems

A one-piece ostomy system is a simple device that combines the pouch and adhesive barrier into a single element. Here's what you should know about this kind of system.

- Ease of Use: Because there is only one component to apply, one-piece systems are usually simple to use and quick to replace. This might be useful for those who are new to ostomy management or want a simple procedure.
- Inconspicuous Design: One-piece pouches are often smaller and more inconspicuous than two-piece systems, making them a popular option for people who want their appliance to be less visible beneath clothes.
- Limited Flexibility: The disadvantage of a one-piece system is that the complete appliance must be replaced every time, which may result in more frequent wear and tear on the skin around your stoma. Furthermore, if you need to move the barrier without altering the bag, this might be more difficult.

One-piece systems are great for consumers who value simplicity and want a sleek, low-profile design.

2 Piece Systems

A two-piece ostomy system is made consisting of a separate pouch and an adhesive barrier that join together via a coupling device. This sort of system provides greater versatility and personalization, but it may take some work to grasp.

- Customizable Components: The most notable benefit of a two-piece system is the ability to replace the pouch without removing the adhesive barrier. This is especially useful if you need to empty your pouch often while minimizing discomfort to the peristome skin.
- Easier Management: Two-piece systems enable you to replace the pouch more often than the barrier, extending the adhesive's lift and lowering the risk of skin irritation. You may also choose various pouch sizes based on your requirements—smaller pouches for short excursions and bigger bags for overnight usage.
- Somewhat Bulkier: Two-piece systems may be somewhat bulkier than one-piece systems due to the presence of two components. However, technological advancements have made these systems much more subtle than they formerly were.

Many patients feel that two-piece systems provide them more flexibility and control over their stoma care regimen, which leads to increased comfort and adaptability.

3. Drainable and Closed Pouches

In addition to choose whether to use a one-piece or two-piece system, you must also choose the kind of pouch that best matches your stoma output and routine:

- Drainable Pouches: These pouches are intended to be drained when full, rather than removed and replaced. They feature an unsealed aperture at the bottom that allows the contents to drain into the toilet. Drainable pouches are appropriate for persons with frequent output since they need less frequent replacement. Most drainable pouches have a secure sealing method to avoid leakage.
- Closed Pouches: Closed pouches, as the name implies, are sealed and designed to be thrown after one usage. These pouches are appropriate for folks with less regular output or who want a more straightforward disposal approach. Closed pouches may need to be changed multiple times each day, but they are ideal for short-term usage, such as when traveling or at special events.

Your output frequency, lifestyle, and personal preferences will determine whether you use drainable or closed pouches. Some individuals like to keep both sorts on hand for usage in various scenarios.

Various Barriers and Adhesive Materials

The adhesive barrier is an essential component of the ostomy equipment, since it forms a seal over the stoma and protects the surrounding skin. It attaches the pouch to your body, and selecting the appropriate barrier is critical for minimizing leaks and keeping healthy skin.

There are a variety of barriers and adhesive materials to consider:

1. Flat and Convex Barriers

The design of the adhesive barrier determines how well the device fits around your stoma.

- Flat Barriers: These barriers lie flat against the skin and are ideal for stomas that protrude slightly from the belly. Flat barriers are ideal for those with even skin contours around the stoma. They're a suitable alternative if your stoma is slightly above the skin's surface (known as a "normal" or "outward" stoma).

- Convex Barriers: Convex barriers have a tiny curvature that pushes the stoma outward, resulting in a tighter fit for stomas that are recessed (below the skin surface) or flush with the skin. These barriers assist to avoid leaks by ensuring that the stoma output goes straight into the pouch rather than leaking beneath the glue. Convex barriers may help support uneven or delicate abdomen skin.

If you are experiencing leaks or skin discomfort, switching to a convex barrier may assist establish a more secure seal. Many patients consult with their stoma nurse to choose the appropriate barrier form.

2. Standard-Wear and Extended-Wear Barriers

The sort of glue used in the barrier will affect how long it may last before having to be replaced.

- Standard-Wear Barriers: These barriers are best suited for those with thicker, more shaped output. Standard-wear barriers are intended for shorter wear intervals and are often used by people who have a colostomy, since their feces is more solid and less prone to break down the adhesive rapidly.

- Extended Wear Barriers: Extended-wear barriers are intended for extended wear durations and increased durability. These barriers are more resistant to moisture and are good for patients who have an ileostomy or urostomy, since the output is more liquid and normal adhesives break down faster. Extended-wear barriers provide better leak protection and may often be worn for many days at a time.

If you have frequent output or find that your barrier wears down too soon, an extended-wear barrier may be the best option for you.

Choosing the Proper Adhesive Material

In addition to choosing the appropriate barrier form and wear duration, you must pick an adhesive substance that is compatible with your skin type. Ostomy barriers are built of a range of materials, each with its own advantages.

- ⊖ Hydrocolloid Adhesives: The majority of ostomy barriers are constructed of skin-friendly hydrocolloid polymers that absorb moisture to form a seal. Hydrocolloid adhesives expand somewhat when exposed to moisture, forming a secure barrier around the stoma. These adhesives are mild on the skin, making them excellent for persons with sensitive skin or a history of discomfort.

- ⊖ Silicone-Based Adhesives: Silicone-based adhesives are an ideal solution for people with very sensitive skin or hydrocolloid allergies. These adhesives are mild, breathable, and easily removed without causing skin damage. Silicone adhesives are often utilized in specialized stoma care solutions for patients with sensitive skin.

Selecting the appropriate adhesive is critical for avoiding discomfort and ensuring that your gadget remains firmly in place. If you have skin irritation or frequent leaks, speak with your stoma nurse to determine the best adhesive material for your requirements.

How to Change an Ostomy Bag: A Step-by-Step Guide

Changing your ostomy bag is an important aspect of ostomy care. Whether you're new to ostomy care or have been living with a stoma for years, establishing this routine can make you feel more in control and confident in your everyday activities.

Changing an ostomy bag might be scary at first, but with the correct equipment, skills, and experience, the operation becomes manageable and efficient.

Before you begin: gather your supplies

To guarantee a seamless and stress-free bag swap, have all of your materials ready before you begin. Here's a checklist of everything you'll need:

1. New ostomy bag and adhesive barrier (one-piece or two-piece system, depending on which you use)
2. Adhesive remover (optional but useful for carefully removing the previous barrier without damaging your skin)
3. Soft washcloth or gauze pads (for cleaning the area surrounding the stoma).
4. Mild, unscented soap (avoid strong chemicals or lotions that might irritate the skin).
5. Warm water (to clean the region around the stoma)
6. Towel (to dry the skin after cleansing).
7. Stoma powder (optional, if necessary to reduce skin irritation)
8. Barrier ring or paste (to provide a better seal around your stoma, if necessary)
9. Disposable plastic bag (to dump the discarded bag and materials)
10. Hand sanitizer (to ensure cleanliness before and after the change)

Once you've put out all of your supplies, properly clean your hands to reduce the danger of infection.

A Step-by-Step Guide for Changing an Ostomy Bag

Step 1: Preparing Your Work Area: Locate a clean, well-lit area where you may change your luggage comfortably. It is advisable to change your ostomy bag while sitting or standing in front of a mirror, particularly at first, to ensure that your stoma is plainly visible. Spread out a towel or paper towels to provide a clean area for your goods.

Step 2: Remove the old ostomy bag: Peel the sticky barrier away from your skin slowly, beginning at the top and working your way down. Take your time to avoid harming the skin around the stoma. To make this procedure simpler and less irritating to the skin, use an adhesive remover spray or wipe.

If your bag is full, dump it into the toilet first to prevent spillage. Remove the old bag and put it in a disposable plastic bag for appropriate disposal.

Step 3: Clean the Skin around the Stoma: Use warm water and a soft washcloth or gauze to gently clean the skin surrounding your stoma. You may use mild, unscented soap, but avoid products with additional scents or lotions, since these might irritate the skin and make it difficult for the adhesive to adhere. Make careful to clean any discharge that has come into touch with the skin.

After cleansing, carefully dry the area with a soft cloth or gauze pad. Ensuring that your skin is totally dry will help the new adhesive barrier adhere better.

Step 4: Inspect the Stoma: Take a minute to examine your stoma and the surrounding skin. Your stoma should be pink or red, wet, and round or oval-shaped. If you detect any changes, such as discoloration, bleeding, or unusual swelling, you should contact your healthcare professional. Examine the skin surrounding the stoma for any symptoms of irritation, redness, or rashes, which may signal the need for a new kind of barrier or stoma care regimen.

Step 5: Apply Skin Protection (As needed): If the area surrounding your stoma is prone to irritation, use stoma powder to absorb excess moisture and protect the skin. Apply a tiny quantity of powder on the stoma and brush off any excess. If you're using a barrier ring or paste to provide further skin protection, use it now to form a tight seal around your stoma.

Step 6: Preparing the New Ostomy Bag and Barrier: If you're using a two-piece system, apply the adhesive barrier to your skin before connecting the fresh pouch. For one-piece systems, the pouch and barrier will be used simultaneously. Make sure the adhesive barrier's aperture is the same size and shape as your stoma. If required, use scissors to trim the aperture to accommodate your stoma appropriately. The barrier should fit tightly around the stoma without being too tight.

If the size of your stoma has changed, you should adjust the aperture to minimize discomfort.

Step 7: Attach the new ostomy bag: Once the adhesive barrier is ready, gently line it with your stoma and push firmly against your skin. If you're utilizing a two-piece system, then connect the pouch to the barrier. To ensure a secure seal, push along the edges of the barrier.

Take your time to ensure that the adhesive is free of wrinkles and gaps, which might create leaks. Apply mild pressure to smooth out any wrinkles and ensure the bag is firmly fastened.

Step 8: Ensure Proper Fit and Seal: After attaching the ostomy bag, double-check that everything is correctly aligned and sealed. Run your fingertips over the borders of the sticky barrier to ensure a secure fit. Some individuals like to warm the barrier with their hands for a few minutes before applying it to the skin, which helps the adhesive attach better.

Step 9: Discard the Used Bag and Supplies: Once the new ostomy bag is in place, put the old one, adhesive barrier, and any spent materials in a plastic garbage bag and seal it. It may be disposed of in the garbage. Make care to properly wash your hands after finishing the operation.

Step 10: Wash your hands: Good cleanliness is essential in any medical care regimen. Finally, wash your hands with soap and water.

How often should you change your ostomy bag?

The frequency of ostomy bag changes may vary based on the device you're using and your specific requirements. Here are some broad principles for determining when to replace your ostomy bag:

- One-piece systems: These should be replaced every 1-3 days. Because the sticky barrier is an integral element of the bag, the complete appliance is removed and changed more regularly.
- Two-piece systems: Two-piece systems allow you to change the bag without having to replace the adhesive barrier as often. The barrier should be changed every 3-4 days, however the bag may be emptied and replaced as required.

When Is It Time for a Change?

Knowing when to replace your ostomy bag is essential for preserving comfort and preventing leaks or discomfort. Here are some indicators that it's time for a change.

- Discomfort or itchiness: If you get itchy, uncomfortable, or detect any irritation around the stoma, it may be time to replace the adhesive barrier.
- Noticing bulging or fullness: If your ostomy pouch feels full or heavy, it's time to empty or replace it. Waiting too long might result in leaking, causing skin discomfort or humiliation.
- Leaking around the edges: If you detect any leaks around the borders of the adhesive barrier, replace your bag right once to prevent skin harm.
- Odor: If you smell a strange odor from the bag, it might mean that the seal around the stoma has been damaged and it's time for a replacement.
- Barrier wear and tear: If the adhesive barrier seems worn or begins to pull away from your skin, replace it before it causes a leak.

Listening to your body and creating a regular shifting schedule will help you keep a habit that works for you while avoiding difficulties.

Changing your ostomy bag becomes second nature with time. While the procedure may seem intimidating at first, following these steps and preparing with the necessary tools can help you feel secure and in charge. Whether you use a one-piece or two-piece system, the key to good ostomy care is understanding when and how to replace your appliance, monitoring the state of your stoma, and maintaining healthy skin surrounding it.

For novices, it might be beneficial to consult with your stoma nurse or healthcare practitioner to verify you're utilizing the appropriate products and practices. With experience, you will develop a regimen that meets your requirements and allows you to live peacefully with your ostomy.

Handling Leaks and Skin Irritation: A Complete Guide

Living with an ostomy requires a learning curve, with one of the most prevalent issues being leaks and skin irritation. While leaks and skin problems may be aggravating, recognizing the reasons and developing a sound preventative and treatment strategy will help you reduce these concerns.

Why Leaks Happen and How to Prevent Them

Leaks may occur for a variety of reasons, but the good news is that many of these causes are preventable with the appropriate tactics. Let's look at the primary sources of leaks and how to avoid them effectively:

1. **Inadequate fit of ostomy appliance**

   - Cause: One of the most prevalent causes of leaking is when an ostomy device does not fit correctly around the stoma. If the adhesive barrier does not form a tight seal, output may leak beneath it and irritate the skin.
   - Prevention: Regularly measure your stoma, particularly in the first few months following surgery, since its size might alter. Cut the aperture in the barrier to match the size of your stoma using a measuring guide (manufacturers typically give these). The fit should be snug but not too tight.

2. **Stoma form or Size Changes**

   - Cause: Weight fluctuations, surgical recuperation, or natural changes might cause your stoma to alter form or size over time. A once-perfect fit might become too loose or tight, resulting in leaks.
   - Prevention: If your stoma changes form or size, modify the aperture of your ostomy barrier to match. You may need to switch to a different product, such as a convex barrier, which offers greater adherence for recessed or irregularly shaped stomas. Consult your stoma nurse to verify you're using the proper sort of barrier.

3. Moisture on the Skin

   - Cause: Moist skin may prevent the adhesive barrier from adhering effectively, resulting in leaks.
   - Prevention: After cleansing your skin, ensure that it is totally dry before inserting a new ostomy equipment. Using a soft cloth or gauze, gently massage the area surrounding your stoma dry. If you

have naturally oily or sweaty skin, try applying an adhesive skin prep or barrier wipe to assist the adhesive adhere more effectively to your skin.

4. Excessive Movement or Activity

- Cause: Physical activity, such as bending or straining, may cause the adhesive barrier to lift off the skin, leading to leaks.
- Prevention: Use ostomy belts or adhesive strips for more security, particularly if you intend to participate in strenuous activity. You may also benefit from utilizing a more flexible device that moves with your body.

5. Gas buildup in the pouch

- Cause: Ostomy bags may fill with gas (known as "ballooning"), placing strain on the seal and resulting in leakage.
- Prevention: Choose a pouch with a built-in filter to assist expel gas while preventing smells from escaping. If ballooning is a common issue, avoid items that produce gas and take the time to "burp" the pouch as needed.

6. Improper Barrier Adhesion

- Cause: Poor ostomy barrier adhesion may be caused by applying the incorrect adhesive or improperly fastening it
- Prevention: Use ostomy-specific adhesives and follow the manufacturer's application directions. If the barrier does not adhere adequately, consider applying an adhesive barrier ring, paste, or spray for further security.

Managing Minor Skin Irritation

Even with a carefully applied appliance, skin discomfort might develop. Minor irritations are frequent and treatable if caught early.

1. Causes of Skin Irritation

- Leaks: Output from the stoma may cause irritation, redness, or pain to the skin surrounding it.
- Frequent Changes: Constantly removing and reapplying adhesive barriers may cause friction, making the skin uncomfortable or injured.
- Sensitive Reactions: Some persons may be sensitive to the components included in ostomy equipment or adhesives.

2. How to Manage Minor area Irritation:

Gently wipe the area surrounding the stoma with warm water and a soft towel. Avoid using strong soaps or chemicals, which may dry out or irritate the skin.

- Use Stoma Powder: If the skin surrounding your stoma is sore or weepy, stoma powder may assist absorb moisture while also protecting it. Before applying a fresh barrier, lightly sprinkle the affected region with stoma powder and remove any excess.
- Barrier Creams and Wipes: Barrier creams or wipes may assist provide a barrier between your skin and the adhesive. These solutions keep your skin safe from irritation while enabling the adhesive to adhere firmly.
- Give Your Skin Time to Heal: If feasible, let your skin "breathe" in between changes. Avoid over tightening the barrier, since this may create further discomfort.

3. When to Seek Medical Treatment for Skin Irritation

If your skin irritation does not improve with simple treatment or worsens (for example, open sores, extreme redness, swelling), contact your stoma nurse or healthcare professional. They may offer other goods or treatments, or they may look for underlying problems like infections.

Choosing Protective Products, such as Skin Barriers and Powders

Choosing the appropriate protective products for your skin type and lifestyle is essential for preserving healthy skin around the stoma. Here are some choices to consider:

1. Skin Barriers (Wafers)

- Purpose: Skin barriers protect the skin surrounding your stoma and provide a tight seal between your appliance and skin.
- Types: Skin barriers exist in a variety of shapes, including flat and convex, and with or without adhesive backing. Depending on the size of your stoma, you may choose between pre-cut or cut-to-fit solutions.
- Choosing the Right Barrier: If your stoma is flush or recessed, a convex barrier might assist you achieve a more secure seal. If your skin is prone to irritation, try using a barrier with skin-soothing components like aloe-vera or vitamin E.

Barrier rings and stripes bridge gaps between skin and adhesive barrier to prevent leakage.

- Apply the barrier ring to your stoma before applying your ostomy device. These items are appropriate for those who have irregular stomachs or uneven skin surfaces.
- How to Choose the Right Ring: Some barrier rings are thicker or more malleable than others, so try out several varieties to see which one works best for your skin and stoma shape.

3. Stoma Powder

To control and protect damp or irritated skin at the stomach. It absorbs excess moisture, avoiding more skin damage.

- How to Use: Apply stoma powder to itchy or damp skin, then brush away any excess. Then, use a barrier wipe to "seal" the powder before applying your ostomy barrier on top.
- Choosing the Right Powder: Most stoma powders are formulated for delicate skin and are devoid of perfumes and harsh chemicals. If you are having problems finding a powder that is suitable for your skin, speak with your stoma nurse.

4. Barrier Wipes and Sprays

- Purpose: These wipes or sprays provide a thin protective barrier on the skin, shielding it from adhesives and stomas.

- Use Instructions: Wipe or spray the product over clean, dry skin before applying your ostomy barrier. Allow the product to dry fully before adding the ostomy equipment.
- How to Choose the Right Product: Some barrier wipes include substances such as aloe or vitamins to help soothe sensitive skin. If your skin is easily irritated, seek for hypoallergenic cosmetics.

Tips for Handling Leaks and Irritations

- Maintain a Regular Changing Schedule: Follow a plan for changing your ostomy device, even if it seems to be operating well. This helps to reduce leaks and skin discomfort
- Avoid Irritating meals: Certain meals might cause more watery output or gas, increasing the likelihood of leaks. Keep a food journal to see which items cause issues and alter your diet appropriately
- Stay Hydrated: Drinking adequate water keeps your stoma output moderate and avoids dehydration, which may result in thicker output that is more difficult to regulate
- Consult Your Stoma Nurse: Your stoma nurse is a great source for product suggestions, hints, and information on how to manage leaks and skin irritation. If you are experiencing persistent problems, do not hesitate to seek expert help.

Best Practices for Odor Management: A Practical Guide to Ostomy Care

One of the most prevalent concerns for ostomy patients is controlling stoma smell. While odor control may seem to be a difficult endeavor, with the correct tactics, it is extremely possible.

Understanding the Causes of Odor

Odor from an ostomy pouch is often created by the digestive process, when specific foods and microorganisms degrade in the body. Some meals naturally generate more gas and greater odors, but others might help minimize odor. Fortunately, new ostomy pouches are made of odor-proof fabrics, which means that the majority of the stench is confined inside the pouch until you empty it. However, controlling the items you consume and using the correct products may help to lessen odor.

Foods that may produce odors

While everyone's digestive system reacts differently to food, certain meals are renowned for producing greater smells in the stool or gas in the pouch. Here's a list of common odor-causing foods:

1. Cruciferous Vegetables

Examples include broccoli, cauliflower, cabbage, and Brussels sprouts.
- Why Do They Cause Odor: These plants contain sulfur compounds, which may produce a strong odor when digested.

2. Why Onions and Garlic Cause Odor:

Onions and garlic are rich in sulfur, which not only provides flavor to your meals but also causes gas and pungent odors during digestion.

3. Fish:

When fish, particularly oily species such as salmon and tuna, are digested, they may produce a strong odor. It may remain in the ostomy pouch after meals.

4. Why Eggs Cause Odor

Eggs are another sulfur-containing item that may produce strong odors after consumption.

5. Why Do Spicy Foods Cause Odor:

Spices, particularly curries and spicy peppers, may contribute to a more pungent odor owing to their strength and interaction with the digestive system.

6. Dairy Products:

Examples include milk, cheese, and yogurt.

- Why Do They Cause Odor: Lactose intolerant or dairy sensitive persons may have increased flatulence and strong-smelling output after ingesting these goods.

7. **Why Do Beans and Lentils Cause Odor**:

These beans contain strong fiber and may create gas during digestion, which increases odor in the ostomy pouch.

Odor-Neutralizing Foods

Some meals generate odor, while others assist to neutralize it. Including these items in your diet may help reduce unpleasant odors:

1. Parsley: Parsley, known for its inherent deodorizing capabilities, may help neutralize the odors of other meals.

2. Yogurt (with living cultures): Yogurt with probiotics may improve digestion and decrease gas and odor.

3. The Benefits of Cranberry Juice: Cranberry juice may help neutralize odors in the digestive system. Some patients report that it decreases odor in their ostomy output.

4. How Buttermilk Can Help: Buttermilk, like yogurt, includes active cultures that aid digestion and decrease gas, which may help minimize odors.

5. Mint: Including mint in your diet, whether as a tea or by chewing fresh mint leaves, may help eliminate odors.

6. Tomatoes: Tomatoes are inherently acidic, which may help balance the pH in your digestive tract and reduce odor.

Odor-Neutralizing Products and Sprays

In addition to regulating your diet, there are many odor-neutralizing items available to help you feel confident throughout the day. Here are some frequent choices:

1. Deodorizing Drops: Deodorizing drops are used in the ostomy pouch to eliminate odors from inside. They are a discreet and easy choice for everyday usage.
   - How to use them: Every time you change or empty your ostomy pouch, place a few drops inside. The drops will work to neutralize smells all day.

2. Odor-Reducing Tablets: Odor-reducing pills are oral supplements that are taken with food. These serve to minimize gas and stink from inside the digestive tract, preventing odor before it occurs.
   - How to Use them: As directed by the manufacturer, take the prescribed dose with meals.

3. Odor-Neutralizing Sprays: These sprays are supposed to be applied around your pouch after emptying it. They eliminate smells that escape during the emptying procedure.
   - How to Use them: To minimize residual odors, spray a little mist over the room or straight into the pouch after emptying.

4. Charcoal Filters: Charcoal filters in ostomy pouches filter out gas while preventing odor release.
   - How to Use them: If your present pouch system does not have a filter, you may buy filters that adhere to your pouch. These enable gas to exit with little scent, which reduces ballooning and stink problems.

5. Pouch Odor-Sealing Technology: Most current ostomy pouches use odor-proof materials to prevent odors from escaping. Use a high-quality bag to offer maximum protection.
   - How to Use It: Make sure your bag is well packed and replace it on a regular basis to prevent odors from previous output.

Discreet Disposal Tip

Another part of odor control is the disposal of old ostomy pouches. Dispose of your bag discreetly to protect privacy and reduce residual odors. Here are some suggestions for controlling disposal:

1. Double Bagging: Place the used ostomy pouch in a tiny, sealable plastic bag, then dispose of it in a separate bag before tossing it away. Double bagging helps to control smells and keeps the pouch from leaking.
- Where to Find Bags: Many ostomy companies sell tiny disposal bags with tight seals. Alternatively, you might use compact, sealable food storage bags.

2. Using Scented Trash Bags: Using scented trash bags may help conceal odors when disposing of pouches in conventional trash cans. The perfume from the bag will assist to mask any possible odors.
- How to Use them: Simply insert the double-bagged pouch in the scented trash bag and dispose of it normally.

3. Use a Dedicated Bin: If feasible, have a small, dedicated trash container in the bathroom for disposing of ostomy items. To help restrict odors, line the bin with scented garbage bags or use an airtight container with a cover.
- How to Manage the Bin: To maintain the bin fresh, empty it on a regular basis to prevent stench buildup, and clean it on occasion using mild soap and water.

4. Deodorizing Trash Spray: Spraying deodorizer into the trash bin before inserting your old pouch will assist neutralize odors when disposing of the pouch.
- How to Use It: Lightly spritz the interior of the bin after each disposal or after replacing the garbage bag.

5. Flushable Liners: Certain ostomy systems have flushable liners that go within the pouch. After usage, the liner may be removed and flushed down the toilet, eliminating the need to dispose of the whole pouch.
- How to use them: Replace the flushable lining whenever you empty your bag. Before utilizing this option, ensure that your plumbing system is capable of handling flushable materials.

Extra Tips for Managing Odor

1. Empty the pouch regularly: Do not wait until your ostomy pouch is entirely filled before emptying it. A filled pouch allows odors to escape, increasing the likelihood of leaks. Empty your bag when it is one-third to halfway fill.

2. Clean the Tail of the Pouch: After emptying your pouch, properly clean the tail or aperture with toilet paper or a baby wipe to prevent lingering odor upon re-sealing.

3. Stay Hydrated: Drinking enough of water helps keep your digestive system functioning and reduces the severity of odors. Staying hydrated also prevents constipation and keeps your output manageable.

Part 5: Nutrition and Dietary Changes

How an Ostomy Affects Digestion: Understanding the New Normal

Your digestive process will be somewhat changed after ostomy surgery, whether it is a colostomy, ileostomy, or urostomy. This chapter will help you understand how your ostomy impacts digestion, what changes to anticipate, and how to adjust your diet to maintain maximum health and comfort. It is understandable to have concerns about food choices, digestion, and how the ostomy may affect your lifestyle.

Digestive Changes Depending on the Type of Ostomy

Each form of ostomy—colostomy, ileostomy, or urostomy—has a unique influence on digestion because it changes the body's normal waste-handling function.

1. Colostomy

A colostomy involves diverting a part of the colon to form a stoma, which allows waste to travel through the stoma rather than the rectum. Depending on where the stoma is located throughout the colon, digestion may be impaired to varied degrees.
- Sigmoid Colostomy (Lower Colon): If the colostomy is located in the sigmoid or descending colon, most of the water has been

absorbed by the waste before it reaches the stoma. Stool is more solid, and digestion mimics normal bowel function. Dietary adjustments may be minor in this scenario.
- Ascending or Transverse Colostomy (Upper Colon): When the stoma is located further up, such as in the transverse or ascending colon, the feces may be softer or semi-formed due to less time for water absorption. You may notice a need for further dietary modifications to assist regulate output consistency.

2. Ileostomy

An ileostomy diverts the small intestine (ileum) to produce the stoma, completely bypassing the colon. This has a greater influence on digestion since the colon is important for absorbing water and nutrients. With an ileostomy, output is usually more liquid and frequent, therefore you have to:
- Stay hydrated: As the colon is skipped, the body loses more water, making dehydration a major issue.
- Nutritional Absorption: Because nutrients are mostly absorbed in the small intestine, an ileostomy may lead to shortages if not properly controlled. Foods high in electrolytes, vitamins, and minerals become essential.

3. Urostomy

A urostomy differs from earlier varieties in that it diverts pee rather than feces. The digestive system is generally intact; nevertheless, dietary adjustments may be required to avoid urinary tract infections or regulate fluid intake.

How Different Foods Affect Stoma Output

After ostomy surgery, your body's reaction to food may change from before. Certain meals might produce changes in your output, such as increased gas, odor, thicker or thinner consistency, or even frequency variations. Understanding how various foods affect your stoma might give you greater confidence when making dietary decisions.

1. Fiber-rich Foods

High-fiber foods, such as fruits, vegetables, whole grains, and legumes, aid digestion. However, if you've had an ileostomy or colostomy, consuming high-fiber meals may cause blockages or excess gas.

- Impact on Stoma Output: Fiber may thicken stool, which may benefit people who have watery output. However, consuming significant quantities fast might result in obstructions. Introduce fiber carefully into your diet and avoid foods that are difficult to digest, such as raw vegetables, maize, and nuts, particularly in the first few weeks after surgery
- Best Practices: When consuming high-fiber meals, chew carefully and remain hydrated to avoid difficulties. Choose cooked vegetables or peeled fruits first, since they are simpler to digest.

2. Hydration and electrolytes

Water and electrolyte balance is particularly important for ileostomy patients since the colon's water-absorbing function is bypassed.

- The Effect on Stoma Output: If you don't drink enough water, your stool may thicken, and you may feel tired or have dehydration symptoms like dizziness or headache. Low electrolyte levels (sodium, potassium) may also develop, causing abnormalities in your general health.
- Best Practice**: Drink lots of fluids, including electrolyte-rich liquids like coconut water or oral rehydration treatments if necessary. Bananas (high in potassium) and broth-based soups (heavy in salt) may assist maintain equilibrium.

3. Protein-rich foods

Following surgery, your body needs more protein to mend tissues and preserve muscle mass. However, protein foods such as red meat might sometimes result in thicker output and harsher odors.

- The Effect on Stoma Output: While protein is necessary for healing, some types, especially fatty portions of meat, might produce increased gas and bulkier stool. Eggs, fish, and lean meats are great protein sources that do not cause substantial difficulties.
- Best Practice: Incorporate lean protein sources and monitor how your body reacts. Chew properly and avoid eating huge quantities in one sitting to help digestion.

4. Fat or Greasy Foods

Fried or oily meals may be more difficult to digest for those with ostomies, especially ileostomies.

- The Effect on Stoma Output: These meals might result in watery or loose output because the fat is not as effectively absorbed. This might be especially difficult if you already suffer with hydration.
- Best Practice: Limit your consumption of fried foods and instead choose healthy fats such as avocados, almonds, and olive oil. These choices are easy to digest and provide necessary nutrients.

5. Gas-producing foods

Gas may cause discomfort and bloating of the ostomy pouch. Certain meals are known for causing gas, such as

- Examples include beans, fizzy beverages, onions, cabbage, and chewing gum.
- Impact on Stoma Output: Gas may cause pain, frequent pouch emptying, and possibly humiliation owing to odor.
- Best Practice: Identify foods that cause you to have excess gas and eat them in moderation. You might also try eating smaller meals throughout the day to avoid gas buildup.

6. Foods to Thicken Output

If your stool is too watery or frequent, some meals might help thicken it and offer you greater control over your bowel movements.

- Examples include applesauce, bananas, peanut butter, bread, rice, and potatoes.
- Effect on Stoma Output: These meals are often suggested if your output is watery or loose. They may decrease digestion and increase consistency.
- Best Practice: Incorporate these meals gradually to evaluate how they affect your productivity. Keep a meal journal to see which items assist thicken your production.

7. Foods That Loosen Production

Sometimes you have difficulties passing stool, or your output becomes excessively thick. In such circumstances, introducing certain meals may assist.

- EXAMPLES: Prune juice, leafy greens, and fruits such as pears and plums.
- Impact on Stoma Output: These meals serve as natural laxatives, softening the stool and making digestion simpler.
- Best Practice: Use these foods sparingly, since they may cause watery output. Drink lots of water to stay hydrated.

When I had my ileostomy surgery, one of the most difficult changes was determining how my new body would react to food. Before surgery, I never considered how various meals may affect my digestion in such particular ways. I'll never forget the first time I ate a bowl of my favorite broccoli soup—something I enjoyed before surgery—and was faced with severe gas and inflating in my pouch. It was a humbling experience.

However, it wasn't long before I began maintaining a food journal. I created a list of which meals generated gas, which thickened or loosened my output, and which I could still eat without problems. I slowly started to feel more in control. I discovered that bananas were my go-to when things were overly liquid, and that chewing my meals thoroughly helped avoid clogs. One of the greatest surprises? The benefits of being hydrated. I'd always drunk water throughout the day, but following the operation, I realized I needed to drink a lot more to keep my body operating correctly. Coconut water was a lifeline for me.

By experimenting and paying careful attention to how my body reacted, I gradually regained my confidence in eating. Now, I can eat a wide range of meals without anxiety, all while being conscious of what works best for me.

Staying Hydrated: An Important Part of Ostomy Care

Hydration is necessary for everyone, but it is especially important for ostomates, particularly those with ileostomies, to preserve their health and well-being. Following ostomy surgery, the digestive system's normal functions are changed, which often impairs the body's capacity to absorb water and electrolytes. Understanding how to remain hydrated, identifying indications of dehydration, and controlling electrolyte imbalances are all important aspects of living well with a stoma.

Importance of Fluids for Ostomates

Following ostomy surgery, especially for those with an ileostomy, the colon's role in water and salt absorption is bypassed. This causes greater water loss, placing ileostomates at a higher risk of dehydration than those with a healthy colon. People who have colostomies still need hydration, albeit they may retain more water depending on how much of the colon remains intact. Urostomates, too, must maintain appropriate fluids to avoid urinary tract infections and support their kidneys.

1. How Does the Body Lose Water?

In a typical digestive tract, the colon absorbs a large quantity of the water you consume, which helps to keep stool firm and your body hydrated. With an ileostomy, stool skips the colon, thus considerable water is lost in the outflow, resulting in loose, watery stools. In certain situations, the body might lose more than two liters of fluids every day. This might result in dehydration and electrolyte imbalances if fluid intake is not altered to compensate for these losses.

2. Hydration Requirements of Ostomates

Ileostomates and colostomates both need to drink more fluids than the ordinary individual to compensate for fluid loss. This involves drinking water, electrolyte-rich drinks, and consuming meals high in water content. The objective is to keep the body hydrated enough to promote cellular activity, keep blood pressure stable, and enable the kidneys to efficiently filter waste products.

Water is essential for ostomates to avoid urinary tract infections and keep their kidneys functioning normally. Keeping the urinary system cleansed with water reduces the chance of bacterial accumulation.

What Amount Should You Drink?

Ostomates often need to drink 2.5 to 3 liters (or more) of liquids every day. However, this figure might vary based on environment, exercise intensity, and personal body demands.

- Ileostomy: If you have an ileostomy, you may need to consume more than three liters of water and other fluids per day to compensate for the water loss via the stoma.
- Colostomy: Colostomates may need significantly less hydration, but still more than the average recommended fluid intake for non-ostomates (typically 2 liters).
- Urostomy: People with ostomies should strive for at least 2 liters per day to avoid urinary tract infections and maintain their kidneys working properly.

The color of your urine is one of the most reliable markers of proper hydration; it should be light yellow or clear. Dark yellow or amber urine may indicate that you should increase your hydration intake.

Symptoms of Dehydration and Electrolyte Imbalance

Individuals with ostomies may rapidly develop dehydration and electrolyte imbalances owing to the body's diminished capacity to retain fluids and salts. Knowing the warning signals is critical for addressing the issue early and avoiding problems.

1. Common signs of dehydration

- Dry Mouth and Thirst: One of the first and most visible indicators of dehydration is a dry mouth along with a strong desire to drink water. If you feel constantly thirsty despite drinking, it means you need more fluids.
- Fatigue: Feeling especially fatigued, sluggish, or weak might indicate that your body is dehydrated. Without adequate hydration, your blood volume falls, lowering the effectiveness of your circulatory system.
- Dark Urine: As previously said, dark urine, such as amber or brownish, indicates that your body is dehydrated.
- Dizziness or Lightheadedness: If you feel dizzy or lightheaded, especially while standing up, it might be a sign of dehydration as the body fights to keep blood pressure stable without enough fluid intake.

- Dry Skin and Eyes: Dehydration may cause your skin to lose suppleness, making it dry or flaky. You may also find your eyes are dry and inflamed.
- Headaches: Because the brain is sensitive to fluid loss and decreased blood flow, dehydration often causes headaches.

2 Signs of Electrolyte Imbalance

Electrolytes—minerals including sodium, potassium, and chloride—help your body balance fluids, sustain neuronal function, and promote muscular action. Electrolyte loss from stoma output may produce imbalances in ileostomates, which can progress to more severe symptoms if left untreated.

- Muscular Cramps: A shortage of potassium or salt in the body may lead to severe muscular cramps or spasms. These are frequent signs of electrolyte depletion.
- Confusion or Cognitive Issues: Electrolyte imbalances may disrupt brain function, causing confusion, difficulties focusing, or a sense of "foggy" thinking.
- Heart Palpitations: Irregular heartbeats or palpitations may develop when electrolyte levels, notably potassium and sodium, become low.
- Nausea and Vomiting: Dehydration and electrolyte imbalances may cause nausea, vomiting, or an upset stomach.

Avoiding Dehydration and Electrolyte Imbalance

The good news is that dehydration and electrolyte abnormalities may be treated and avoided with proper fluid and nutritional intake. Here are some practical ways for staying hydrated and maintaining adequate electrolyte levels:

1. Drink little amounts on a regular basis

Rather than drinking big amounts of water all at once, which may travel through your system too rapidly, try to sip it throughout the day. Carry a water bottle with you as a reminder to drink frequently.

2. Use Electrolyte-Rich Fluids

In addition to water, it is critical to replenish lost electrolytes. Drinking drinks with salt, potassium, and other essential minerals may assist. Options include:
- Oral Rehydration Solutions (ORS): Specially made rehydration liquids containing a balanced combination of electrolytes and carbohydrates.
- Coconut Water is naturally high in potassium and a wonderful source of hydration.
- Sports Drinks: These may assist in restoring lost electrolytes, but be wary of the sugar content. If sugar-free or low-sugar alternatives are available, choose these.

3. Consume hydrating foods

Incorporating high-water-content items into your meals will help you meet your daily fluid requirements. Examples include:
- Cucumber: With a water content of around 95%, cucumbers are a good snack for staying hydrated.
- Watermelon: A pleasant and hydrating fruit abundant in water and naturally occurring sugars.
- Tomatoes are high in water and nutrients such as vitamin C.
- Leafy Greens: Vegetables like lettuce and spinach are high in water and hence excellent sources of hydration.

4. Monitor Your Salt Intake

While sodium is sometimes seen as something to avoid, for ostomates, taking the appropriate amount of salt is critical for maintaining electrolyte balance, particularly when coping with significant water loss via stomas. Adding a little salt to your meals or drinking broth will help keep your sodium levels stable.

5. Avoid caffeine and alcohol

Both coffee and alcohol are diuretics, which means they cause your body to lose more water than it takes in. While you don't have to completely avoid them, it's recommended to consume them in moderation and drink plenty of water while drinking coffee, tea, or alcohol.

6. Identify Warning Signs Early

Pay attention to how your body feels. If you observe indications of dehydration or electrolyte imbalance, such as persistent lethargy, dizziness, or dark urine, take quick action to hydrate and replenish electrolytes.

Shortly after my ileostomy surgery, I didn't realize how important water was for my health. One hot summer day, I spent a few hours gardening in the heat. I drank some water, but it wasn't enough to make up for the fluid loss. That evening, I began to feel dizzy and lightheaded, and my lips felt like sandpaper. Worse, I couldn't think clearly; I felt fuzzy and bewildered. I hadn't realized it at the time, but I was getting dangerously dehydrated.

The following morning, I awoke with a pounding headache and saw that my pee was dark, nearly brownish. It was a terrifying time since I had no clue how soon dehydration may strike. Thankfully, after speaking with my healthcare professional, I learned how to properly regulate my hydration. Now, I never leave the home without a water bottle, and I make an effort to incorporate electrolyte-rich liquids in my daily regimen.

That encounter was a wake-up call. It taught me that, although living with an ostomy may be challenging at times, maintaining hydrated and mindful of my body's demands has given me the means to live more easily and confidently.

Part 6: Lifestyle Adjustments and Daily Life

Clothing Choices: Dressing Comfortably and Confidently with an Ostomy

One of the most difficult changes following ostomy surgery might be finding out how to dress comfortably and elegantly while tolerating your stoma and ostomy equipment. The good news is that with a little forethought and the appropriate selections, you can still wear most of your favorite clothing designs. From underwear and swimwear to sporting and formal attire, the goal is to discover what works best for your body and lifestyle.

Living with an ostomy does not imply compromising your unique style. Whether you like casual clothing, fitness gear, or more formal wear, there are several alternatives to make you feel confident and comfortable.

1. General Clothing Tips

After ostomy surgery, it's normal to be anxious about how your pouch will appear beneath your clothing and how to keep it hidden. The key to dressing appropriately with an ostomy is to prioritize comfort while keeping your ostomy appliance secure and unobtrusive.

Loose Fit vs. Form-Fitting Clothing

- -Loose and Flowy Clothing: Loose or flowy clothes are frequently the most comfortable way to wear an ostomy. A-line dresses, baggy blouses, tunics, and wide-leg slacks may assist disguise the pouch while still allowing you to move freely. These types work especially well while you're still adjusting to your stoma and experimenting with what feels best.
- High-Waisted Clothing: High-waisted jeans, skirts, and shorts work well for fastening and concealing the ostomy equipment. They may

hold the bag against your body, making it less noticeable and lowering the possibility of accidental separation.
- Layers: Layering may save your life. Wearing a cardigan, jacket, or over shirt provides an added layer of subtlety while also enabling you to change your comfort based on temperature or activity level.
- Elastic Waistbands: Elastic waistbands in pants, skirts, or shorts are an excellent approach to assure comfort while also accommodating variations in your body size or form, which might vary after surgery. They are very tolerant when your bag starts to fill and needs more space.

Workable Fabrics

- Breathable Fabrics: Use lightweight fabrics such as cotton, linen, or bamboo that enable airflow to keep the region around your stoma cool and dry. Breathable textiles help lessen the likelihood of sweating and discomfort around the stoma.
- Stretch Fabrics: Clothing composed of stretch fabrics like spandex or lycra provides flexibility and comfort while moving or bending. These textiles conform to the contour of your body and ostomy equipment, making them perfect for everyday use.
- Dark Colors and Patterns: Many ostomates prefer darker colors and patterns, which may help conceal any bulging or pouch shapes. They're also useful for concealing unintentional spills or stains while on the run.

2. Underwear and Accessories

Wearing the proper undergarments is critical for comfort and confidence while dealing with an ostomy. There are several types of undergarments created exclusively for ostomates that give additional support for your pouch while keeping it secure against your body.

Ostomy-specific underwear

- Supportive Underwear: Specifically made ostomy underwear often has built-in pouches or bands to keep the device in place and prevent it from moving or tugging. These undergarments may be both discrete and comfy, boosting your confidence as you go about your day.

- High-Waisted Briefs and Boxers: High-waisted briefs or boxers provide good covering and may assist keep the ostomy pouch in place. Many individuals like these alternatives because they keep the bag from hanging freely and distribute weight more evenly.

Accessories for Increased Security

- Ostomy Belts: These are adjustable bands that wrap around your waist and provide extra support for the pouch. They may assist hold your pouch in place during strenuous exercise or when wearing more fitting apparel.
- Waistbands: Ostomy waistbands provide additional security and comfort. They are worn around your midsection to keep the item in place and might be concealed behind your clothing. They come in a variety of sizes and textures, including soft cotton and flexible textiles.

3. Swimwear for an Ostomy

Ostomates often worry about swimwear, but with the correct options, you may still enjoy the beach or pool. Whether you like one-piece suits, bikinis, or swim shorts, there are plenty fashionable and useful alternatives available.

Swimsuit Options for Women

- High-Waisted Bikinis: High-waisted bikini bottoms are ideal for hiding a pouch. They provide coverage, support, and style all at once. Pair with a beautiful bikini top to feel confident and comfortable in the water.
- One-Piece Swimsuits: A one-piece swimsuit provides greater covering and support for the abdomen, making it simpler to hide the pouch. Look for styles with ruching or patterns to help hide the area.
- Tankinis: Tankinis give you the best of both worlds by giving a covering with a long top and the option to wear a separate bottom. The top may be flowing or fitted, depending on your style.

Swimsuit Options for Men

- Swim Trunks: Many men with ostomies prefer higher-waisted swim trunks that give additional covering for the pouch. To improve security, place an ostomy belt beneath your swim trunks.
- Rash Guards: Wearing swim trunks with a rash guard (a fitting swim shirt) might offer additional covering for the pouch and peace of mind when swimming or participating in aquatic activities.

Swimwear Tips

- Adhesive Strips: If you're worried about your pouch becoming loose in the water, try applying waterproof adhesive strips to fix it even further. These strips are simple to install and help keep the flange edges from flaking off due to dampness.
- Empty before Swimming: To limit the danger of leaks and mishaps, empty your ostomy pouch before entering the water. This will make the pouch feel lighter and more pleasant to swim in.

4. Sports and Active wear

Staying active with an ostomy is not only doable, but also recommended. Whether you're hitting the gym, going for a run, or doing yoga, you may discover comfortable sportswear that fits your ostomy needs.

Supportive Athletic Wear

- Compression Gear: Many ostomates find compression shorts, leggings, or shirts useful for keeping their pouch secure when exercising. These garments deliver mild pressure to the region surrounding the stoma, securing the pouch without impeding mobility.
- High-Waisted Leggings and Shorts: Just like regular clothing, high-waisted leggings and shorts are perfect for giving support and concealing the ostomy device. To minimize pain, choose for sporting attire with a wide, elastic waistband.

How to Choose the Right Fabrics

- Moisture-Wicking textiles: Choose moisture-wicking textiles, such as polyester or nylon blends, to help move perspiration away from your skin and reduce the risk of irritation or infection around the stoma. These fabrics are light, breathable, and ideal for high-intensity exercises.
- Stretch Fabrics: Materials that stretch and move with your body are useful for exercises like yoga, Pilates, and strength training. They keep your ostomy pouch tight, no matter how much you move about.

Activities that may need additional support

- Contact Sports: If you participate in contact sports such as soccer or martial arts, consider wearing extra protective clothing over your stoma. Ostomy guards or shields are offered to keep the stoma safe from impact.
- Running or Jumping: Use a supporting ostomy belt or waistband while participating in high-impact activities such as running, jumping, or aerobics. It may assist keep the bag from bouncing about and pushing on the adhesive barrier.

5. Adaptive Clothing Brands and Styles

Several manufacturers specialize in adapting clothes for individuals with medical equipment, such as ostomy appliances. These firms provide garments with inconspicuous openings, additional support, and other features to make dressing with an ostomy simpler.

Brands to look for

- Ostomysecrets: This business sells a variety of undergarments, wraps, and swimsuits made particularly for persons with ostomies. Their products include built-in compartments to keep the ostomy pouch secure.
- Comfizz: Comfizz is a UK-based business that sells ostomy support products including waistbands, undergarments, and wraps. Their goods are intended to be comfy, discrete, and elegant.
- Stealth Belt: Known for their revolutionary ostomy support belts, Stealth Belt provides solutions for everyday use, sports, and even swimming. Their belts enhance stability and comfort, making it simpler to maintain an active lifestyle.

- CUI Wear: CUI Wear specializes in support garments for persons with ostomies and provides a range of goods, including briefs, boxers, and high-waisted trousers, to give support and lessen the risk of hernias.

Physical Activity and Exercise: Leading an Active Life with an Ostomy

One of the most essential lifestyle changes after ostomy surgery is determining the appropriate mix of rest, healing, and physical activity. Many ostomates find it difficult to resume physical activity, particularly when they are worried about how movement will damage their stoma or ostomy pouch. However, physical activity is critical for preserving general health, emotional well-being, and preventing issues such as weight gain or muscular weakening. Engaging in the appropriate workouts may help you recover strength, enhance vitality, and even lower your risk of issues like hernias.

1. Begin Slowly and Build Strength

Following ostomy surgery, your body will need time to recuperate. Whether you have undergone a colostomy, ileostomy, or urostomy, it is critical to gradually resume physical activity. Rushing into vigorous workouts or carrying large things might cause issues such as hernias or stoma strain. It is always advisable to contact your healthcare professional before beginning any new fitness plan, as they may give tailored advice depending on your surgery and general health.

Key Considerations for Beginning Physical Activity

- Enable Adequate Healing Time: Following surgery, you should avoid strenuous physical activity for at least 6 to 8 weeks to enable your body to recover. Take your surgeon's advice and pay attention to how your body feels. It's critical not to overwork oneself during the early recuperation phase.
- Listen to Your Body: The most crucial tip for restarting exercise is to listen to your body. If you experience any discomfort, pain, or odd feelings around your stoma, cease immediately and contact your doctor. Gentle stretching and gentle walking are excellent strategies to get moving without overworking your body.

- Gradually Increase Activity: Once your doctor gives you the go-ahead, start with low-impact workouts like walking or swimming. As you gain strength and endurance, you may progressively raise the intensity of your exercises. Avoid any activities that require heavy lifting or core strain until you have completely healed.
- Stay Hydrated: Ostomates, especially those with an ileostomy, are more likely to get dehydrated. Exercise may further deplete your fluid levels, so drink lots of water before, during, and after physical exercise to stay hydrated and electrolyte balanced.

2. Best Exercises for Ostomates

Physical activity after ostomy surgery does not have to be restricted. Many ostomates effectively participate in a variety of workouts, including competitive sports. The goal is to begin with easy, low-impact exercises that will help you gain stamina and strength without placing too much strain on your abdomen or stoma.

Walking

Walking is one of the safest and most beneficial types of exercise for ostomates, particularly in the early phases of rehabilitation. It is low-impact, simple to practice anywhere, and can be progressively increased in intensity as you gain strength. Walking improves circulation, increases energy levels, and promotes mental health.

- Begin Slowly: Take small walks around your house or neighborhood, gradually increasing the distance and speed over time. If you feel up to it, start with 10-15 minute walks and gradually increase to 30-45 minutes.
- Upright Posture: Be aware of your posture when walking. Keep your back straight and minimally engage your core to maintain proper form. This will allow you to build your abdominal muscles without stressing them.

Swimming

Swimming is another great alternative for ostomates since it is low-impact and puts less strain on their joints and abdominal muscles. The buoyancy of water supports your body weight, allowing you to move freely without straining your stoma or ostomy pouch.

- Secure Your Pouch: Before entering the water, make sure your ostomy pouch is secured with waterproof tape or an ostomy belt. Although most bags are watertight, additional protection may give further piece of mind. Empty your purse before swimming to prevent bulk.
- Choose the Right Environment: Some ostomates prefer to begin by swimming in private pools or with close relatives and friends. Public swimming pools and beaches are also safe, but if you are worried about visibility, high-waisted swimwear or specialist ostomy swim gear might make you feel more at ease.

Yoga and Stretching

Yoga is good for increasing strength, flexibility, and relaxation. Slow, controlled movements in yoga help you rebuild muscular tone while being aware of your body's limits. Gentle stretching exercises may also assist to reduce stiffness and increase mobility.

- Focus on Low-Intensity postures: During your early recuperation, adhere to beginner-level postures that do not require too much twisting or bending at the waist. Poses such as the child's pose, sitting forward bends, and cat-cow stretches are great for increasing flexibility and relieving stress.
- Avoid Core Strain: While yoga may gradually strengthen your core, avoid difficult poses such as planks, boat positions, and inversions until you've regained adequate abdominal strength.

CYCLING

Cycling, whether on a stationary bike or a regular bicycle, delivers a cardiovascular exercise while minimizing pressure on your stoma. It's ideal for maintaining fitness and can be tailored to various degrees of intensity.

- Stationary Biking: A stationary bike is a safer alternative for early recovery since it lowers the danger of falls or accidents. Begin with brief sessions at low resistance, gradually increasing time and resistance as you gain strength.
- Outside riding: When you're ready to go outside riding, ensure your pouch is tight and protected from unexpected bumps. Wear

comfortable, supportive gear, such as high-waisted leggings or cycling shorts, to keep the pouch in place while riding.

3. Core Strengthening to Prevent Hernias

One of the most prevalent worries for ostomates is the danger of having a parastomal hernia, which is an abdominal hernia that develops around the stoma. Hernias may form when the abdominal muscles are weakened by surgery, therefore developing core strength is critical for avoiding this issue. However, you should proceed with care and only begin core activities when you have completely recovered from surgery.

What is a parastomal hernia?

A parastomal hernia occurs when a portion of the intestine pushes through a weak section of the abdominal wall near the stoma. This may result in pain, swelling, and, in certain circumstances, surgical correction. Strengthening the muscles around your stoma provides support and reduces the chance of hernia development.

Guidelines for Safe Core Strengthening

- Start Slowly: After ostomy surgery, core workouts should be performed with caution. Begin with modest motions that stimulate your abdominal muscles without putting undue pressure on your stoma or abdominal region.
- Engage Your Core Lightly: In workouts like walking, yoga, or even sitting activities, gently activating your core muscles may help them recover strength over time without the need for intense, separate motions.
- Avoid Heavy Lifting: Lifting heavy weights or doing activities that put a lot of strain on your abdominal wall, such as sit-ups or crunches, might raise your risk of hernias. Stick to bodyweight workouts that include modest core involvement.

Best Core Exercises for Osteoporosis

1. Pelvic Tilts: Lie on your back, legs bent, and feet flat on the ground. Slowly tilt your pelvis forward, flattening your lower back on the floor, and then let go. This exercise gently stimulates the lower abdominal muscles while avoiding tension.

2. Seated Leg Raises: Sit on a chair, back straight, feet flat on the floor. Lift one leg at a time, keeping it a few inches above the ground for a few seconds before lowering it. This exercise improves lower abdominal strength while maintaining your posture.

3. Bridge Pose: Lie on your back, knees bent, feet hip-width apart. Press your feet into the ground and elevate your hips to form a straight line from your shoulders to your knees. This exercise improves the glutes, lower back, and core muscles.

4. Plank Modifications: Instead of beginning with a complete plank, try modified variants like a forearm plank or a side plank. Hold each posture for a few seconds, keeping your core engaged but without placing too much pressure on your abdomen.

5. Knee-to-Chest Stretch: Lie on your back, legs outstretched. Slowly raise one knee to your chest and hold it with both hands for a few seconds before releasing. This stretch works your lower abs and may improve flexibility.

Use Supportive Gear

- Ostomy or Hernia Belts: Wearing an ostomy or hernia belt while exercising may give extra abdominal support, lowering the risk of hernias. These straps serve to tighten the stoma and prevent it from excessive strain during physical exercise.
- Support Garments: Compression garments or abdominal binders may also aid to support the abdominal muscles and prevent tension during core activities.

4. General Tips for Exercise with an Ostomy

- Empty Your Pouch before Exercise: To minimize pain or leaks during physical exercise, empty your pouch before you begin your workout. This will help you feel lighter and more relaxed.
- Wear the Right Gear: High-waisted or compression sportswear may assist keep your ostomy pouch tight during exercise while also reducing movement and discomfort around the stoma. Look for

- Take Breaks as Needed: Avoid pushing yourself too hard. Rest is an essential aspect of any workout plan, particularly when your body adjusts after surgery. If you experience any pain, dizziness, or weariness, take a rest, drink, and pay attention to your body's cues.
- Stay Hydrated: Dehydration is a worry for ostomates, especially those with ileostomies. Physical activity raises your body's fluid requirements, so stay hydrated before, during, and after exercise. Electrolyte drinks may also assist to restore minerals lost after a lengthy exercise, but see your doctor to confirm they're right for you.
- Communicate with Your Healthcare Team: When beginning or modifying an exercise regimen, always keep your healthcare team informed. They can advise you on which workouts are safe, how to prevent issues like hernias, and how to properly support your stoma during physical activity. Physical therapy may be a safe and effective way for some people to improve their muscles and regain mobility following surgery.

5. Moving Forward: Living an Active Lifestyle with Confidence

Embracing physical exercise following ostomy surgery is not only doable, but also enjoyable and powerful. Many ostomates find that remaining active improves their entire quality of life, with advantages that extend beyond physical health. Exercise promotes mental health, decreases stress, improves mood, and increases energy levels.

You may restore strength, recover confidence, and ultimately return to the activities you like most by starting with baby steps, being attentive of your body's demands, and concentrating on low-impact activities. Whether it's walking, swimming, yoga, or weight training, establishing a regimen that works for you is essential. Over time, your ostomy will most likely become a normal part of your life, rather than something that defines or restricts your skills.

Remember that the aim is not perfection, but development. You may continue an active, healthy lifestyle for many years by gradually building your strength, concentrating on safe workouts, and being aware of your body's signals.

Practical Exercises for Various Fitness Levels

Here are some realistic workout programs geared to the varied fitness levels of ostomates:

The Beginner Routine

- Week 1–2: Begin with 10-15 minutes of walking each day. Concentrate on maintaining excellent posture and a consistent speed. Add mild stretches, such as calf stretches, to improve flexibility.
- Week 3-4: Incorporate mild arm exercises while walking (e.g., arm swings) to work upper body muscles. You may also start exercising your abdominal muscles with simple pelvic tilts and sitting leg lifts.
- Week 5–6: Increase your walking time to 30 minutes. Include 5 minutes of moderate yoga positions like cat-cow, child's pose, and sitting forward folds to enhance flexibility and relieve stress.

The Intermediate Routine

- Week 1–2: Start with 20-30 minutes of brisk walking or stationary cycling. Include mild yoga poses for core and flexibility. Standing postures such as warrior I and II may help you activate your legs and core.
- Week 3-4: Implement mild resistance exercise with resistance bands or small weights. Concentrate on exercises such as sitting rows, bicep curls, and leg extensions. Aim for three sets of 10-12 repetitions for each exercise.
- Week 5-6: Incorporate low-impact aerobic exercises such as swimming or cycling. Core-strengthening exercises like modified planks (on knees) and bridge position should be introduced gradually. Aim for 30-45 minutes of physical exercise, three to four times a week.

Advanced Routine

- Week 1-2: Perform a combination of cardio and strength training, such as 30 minutes of walking followed by 20 minutes of resistance

exercise. Squats, lunges, and push-ups are good examples of whole-body motions.
- Week 3–4: Include core workouts such as side planks and leg lifts. Interval training, which alternates between brisk walking and light running or cycling at varied speeds, may help you increase the intensity of your cardio workouts.
- Week 5-6: Perform more difficult strength workouts using resistance bands or free weights. Concentrate on complex exercises that work several muscle groups, such as squats with overhead presses or lunges with bicep curls. Moderate-intensity cardio exercises should last 45-60 minutes and be done 3-5 times per week.

Traveling with an Ostomy

Travel may be intimidating for anybody, but for those with an ostomy, leaving the security and regularity of home can be especially difficult. However, having an ostomy does not imply abandoning your passion for travel or losing out on life's pleasures. With little planning and preparation, you may comfortably travel to new destinations, whether for a weekend escape, an international vacation, or a work trip.

1. Packing a Travel Kit with Additional Supplies

Having the necessary goods on hand is the first step in preparing for a trip. Whether you're going on a short road trip or a lengthy international journey, carrying a well-organized travel kit ensures you're ready for everything.

Essentials to Pack

Your travel pack should contain everything you'll need for normal stoma care as well as dealing with unforeseen events. Here's a list of things to consider:

- Extra Pouches and Flanges: Carry more than you think you'll need. The basic rule of thumb is to carry twice as much as you would typically use at the same time. If you replace your pouch every two days, bring extra for daily changes just in case
- Barrier Wipes and Powders: These are crucial for keeping your skin irritation-free. Your skin may respond differently in a foreign

environment or when traveling for an extended amount of time, so having them on hand is essential.
- Adhesive Remover: Make sure you have lots of adhesive remover wipes or spray. These are very essential for ensuring that you can remove your ostomy pouch gently, even under stressful conditions.
- Skin Protection Film: Packing a skin protection barrier spray or wipe allows you to reapply it as required while traveling.
- Disposal Bags: It's a good idea to include additional disposable bags to discreetly and hygienically remove spent materials when traveling, particularly on airlines or lengthy road journeys.
- Scissors: If you're using cut-to-fit wafers or flanges, bring a tiny set of travel scissors. Ensure that they follow TSA standards for carry-on goods.
- Hand Sanitizer and Wet Wipes: Stoma care may be challenging in public toilets or under unsanitary settings, so keeping sanitizer and wipes on hand is essential for preserving cleanliness.
- Travel-Sized Spray or Drops for Odor Control: Carry ostomy-specific odor control solutions. A few drops within the bag may help minimize odor, which is especially effective in restricted settings such as aircraft toilets.
- Dry Wipes and Tissues: Dry wipes are required to keep the area around the stoma clean. They are also handy for washing down surfaces in public restrooms.

Organize Your Supplies

It's a good idea to arrange your goods in such a manner that they're conveniently accessible and you can swiftly solve any difficulties without having to fumble through your pack. Use compact pouches or zipped bags to categorize materials (cleaning, changing, and disposal), and make sure your travel kit fits comfortably into your carry-on baggage or personal bag. If you're traveling, carry this kit on you rather than in checked luggage—luggage might be delayed or misplaced, and you need to have access to your supplies at all times.

Always check the weather at your destination and adapt your supplies accordingly. Humidity or heat may affect the adhesive strength of your bag, so carry extra goods or materials appropriate for the area.

2. Navigating Airport Security and Dealing with the TSA

Airports are often a cause of concern for ostomy patients, particularly when it comes to going through security checks. Knowing what to anticipate and planning ahead of time are essential for successfully passing airport security.

Notifying the TSA Officer

When passing through TSA, you are not compelled to notify security about your ostomy, although it may assist make the procedure easier. Many persons with an ostomy prefer to notify the TSA officer before screening starts. You may simply state, "I have a medical device." If you wish to elaborate, tell them that you have an ostomy and may want seclusion or other accommodations. The TSA has mechanisms in place to handle such situations discreetly.

You may also request a private screening if you want to be examined in a different room. The police will most likely do a pat-down and swab the exterior of your ostomy device to detect chemical residue. Rest assured that they will not require you to remove or show your ostomy pouch during screening.

Have a medical note

To make the procedure easier, particularly when traveling overseas, bring a medical certificate or a note from your doctor describing your ostomy. This is optional, however it may assist speed up the procedure if security staff have any queries.

Supplies in your carry-on

As previously said, always bring your goods in your carry-on. The TSA accepts ostomy products such as adhesives, pouches, and barrier wipes in acceptable amounts throughout your travel. These should not be counted against your liquid allowance. If you are worried about having any goods seized, convince the security personnel that they are medically required.

How to Deal with Scanners

Full-body scanners may detect your ostomy pouch, but TSA officials are trained to handle such situations professionally and respectfully. If you are chosen for extra screening, you may request that it be conducted in secret.

Maintain patience and calm during the procedure. TSA officers deal with a wide range of medical ailments and equipment on a regular basis, therefore the majority will be acquainted with ostomies and will offer sufficient discretion.

3. Tips for Long Flights and Road Trips

Long distance travel, whether by air or vehicle, might create unique obstacles for ostomates. Here's how you can make these encounters more pleasant.

Before the Trip

- Eat lightly: The day before you travel, eat lighter meals to lessen the possibility of needing to empty your pouch often.
- Hydrate Well: It's easy to get dehydrated on lengthy excursions, particularly airplanes. Drink lots of water before and during travel, but avoid overconsumption, particularly if toilet access is restricted.

Throughout the Trip

Sit Near the bathroom: If feasible, choose a seat near the bathroom on aircraft or buses. This will relieve worry about having to empty your pouch and make it simpler to handle stoma care discreetly.

- Bring a tiny Pouch of Essentials: If you're going by airline, keep a tiny bag of vital supplies (additional pouches, wipes, barrier cream) in your seatback pocket or a small personal item. This saves you from having to reach for your bigger carry-on bag.
- Empty Your Pouch Before Boarding: Always empty your pouch before boarding a plane or beginning a lengthy road trip. This reduces the likelihood of having to empty it immediately throughout the journey.

For Long Flights

- Remain Hydrated: Airplane cabins are dry, so drink plenty of water to remain hydrated. Be mindful that alcohol and caffeinated drinks might dehydrate you, so try to minimize them.
- Move Around: Take a stroll every hour or so to avoid blood clots and be comfortable. This movement may also aid with digestion.

For Road Trips

- Plan Rest pauses: If you're going by automobile, make frequent pauses to empty your pouch. These stops allow you to stretch and rest, making the ride more enjoyable
- Food Caution: Before you begin your road journey, avoid foods that you know produce gas or stink. This is particularly crucial in restricted areas like as an automobile.

If you're concerned about odor during travel, put odor-neutralizing goods in your pouch before you go. This might provide additional peace of mind while you're on the run.

Many ostomates travel regularly and successfully—your ostomy should be a minor factor in a grand adventure, not a hindrance to your plans.

So pack your luggage, hit the road or the skies, and enjoy your journey knowing you're ready for anything that comes your way.

Managing Work and School with an Ostomy

Living with an ostomy might provide unique obstacles in terms of keeping a typical job or school schedule. Whether you're returning to work, beginning a new career, or taking courses, managing your ostomy requires planning, deliberate decision-making, and knowledge of your rights.

1. Disclose Your Condition (Or Not)

One of the most difficult choices you may have to make following your surgery is whether or not to inform your coworkers, employers, or school personnel about your ostomy. Disclosing your health is a personal decision, with no right or wrong answer—it all depends on what makes you feel comfortable and supported.

To Disclose or Not Disclose?

- The Case for Disclosure: Some people find it beneficial to discuss their ostomy with their boss, human resources (HR) department, or school administrators. Being open about your medical condition may make it simpler to seek accommodations or explain any special requirements, like frequent potty breaks or time off for medical visits. If you work or attend school in a pleasant and supportive environment, openness may develop understanding and decrease the stress of concealing your illness. Disclosing to a trustworthy coworker or classmate might also give extra support if you need it throughout the day.

- The Case for not disclosing: On the other hand, some individuals want to keep their medical issues secret, especially if they feel it will not interfere with their ability to work or go to school. You are not required to reveal your ostomy unless it adversely affects your job or necessitates modifications. If you are uncomfortable discussing your health or are concerned about stigma, it is completely OK to keep the information private and only share it with those who need to know.

How to Disclose Your Ostomy

If you decide to reveal your disease, you should consider how and when to do so. Here are a few suggestions to make the discussion easier:

- Speak with HR or Administration First: If you are worried about your privacy or the reactions of your classmates, consult with your human resources representative or school administration. These specialists are trained to handle medical matters discreetly and may help make arrangements without disclosing unwanted information.

- Keep it Simple: There is no need to go into depth about your ostomy unless you feel comfortable doing so. It can be described as a medical equipment that aids in the management of a health issue, with a concentration on what your supervisor or school authorities need to assist you in succeeding. You may, for instance, state: "I have a medical device that requires me to take occasional breaks to manage it, but it won't affect my ability to complete my work."

- Emphasize Your Needs: The goal of reporting your ostomy is to ensure that you have the appropriate environment and accommodations to flourish. Focus the discussion on any particular requirements you may have, such as more frequent toilet breaks, access to a private restroom, or scheduling flexibility for medical visits.

2. Legal Protections and Accommodations (ADA in the USA)

Individuals with an ostomy in the United States are covered under the Americans with Disabilities Act (ADA), a statute aimed to prevent disability discrimination. Individuals with ostomies are entitled to reasonable accommodations that assist them in managing their condition while at work or school, according to the ADA.

Understanding your rights under the ADA

- What constitutes a "disability" under the ADA?: A disability is defined as any condition that significantly impairs one or more primary living activities. According to this definition, an ostomy is a handicap, which means you are legally protected from discrimination at work or school.
- Reasonable Accommodations: The ADA requires employers and schools to provide reasonable accommodations for people with disabilities, as long as they do not create undue hardship. Reasonable accommodations for ostomates may include:
- Frequent Restroom Breaks: You may need to empty or check your ostomy pouch on a frequent basis. Requesting greater flexibility with breaks is a sensible request.
- Access to a Private toilet: If you feel uncomfortable managing your ostomy in a public toilet, you may request to use a private or staff restroom.

- Adjustments to Your Workstation: If sitting for extended periods of time causes difficulty due to your ostomy, you may request an ergonomic chair or a standing desk.
- Flexible Hours: Some people need to arrange time off for medical appointments or have a modified work schedule. The American Disability Act also offers freedom in this area.

How to Request Accommodations

If you need particular accommodations at work or school, the easiest method to seek them is to speak with HR, your supervisor, or your school's disability services office. Take these steps:

1. Document Your Needs: Before asking your employer or school, consider what particular modifications you need. Consider how your ostomy impacts your daily routine and what changes might make it simpler to manage.

2. Produce Medical Documentation: You may need to produce a doctor's letter describing your medical condition and the accommodations you need. This helps to formalize your request and ensures that your employer or school knows your requirements.

3. Discuss Reasonable Solutions: During your chat, be upfront about your needs while still being flexible. For example, if you're requesting additional toilet breaks, argue that they might be included into your schedule without affecting productivity.

3. Create a Comfortable Environment

Once you've reported your illness and sought accommodations (if necessary), you should consider how to establish a pleasant, supportive atmosphere in which you may manage your ostomy discreetly while remaining focused on your job or studies.

Create a Private and Hygienic Space

Access to a secluded, clean, and pleasant toilet is essential for ostomates at work or school. While many persons with ostomies may use conventional public bathrooms, it's beneficial to have a few procedures in place to make the experience more comfortable:

- Identify facilities with Privacy: If feasible, seek out facilities that provide greater privacy, such as single-stall bathrooms or staff restrooms. These are great for ostomy care since they provide enough room and time to replace or empty your pouch discreetly.
- Keep a Supply Kit Handy: Consider having a small supply kit on your desk or in your locker. This pack may contain additional pouches, adhesive wipes, barrier cream, dry wipes, and disposal bags, ensuring that you are always prepared in the event of an unforeseen leak or need for a change.
- Try Odor Control Products: If you're worried about odor while changing or emptying your pouch at work or school, try odor-neutralizing drops or sprays made specifically for ostomates. These items promote discretion, particularly in communal toilets.

Clothes for Comfort and Confidence

Choosing the appropriate apparel may significantly improve your comfort at work or school. Many ostomates discover that certain designs and materials hide the pouch while giving comfort throughout the day.

- Loose-Fitting Clothes: Choose clothes that do not cling too tightly to your belly, particularly around your stoma. Flowy blouses, high-waisted leggings, and skirts may assist to disguise your ostomy bag and reduce discomfort.
- Supportive Garments: If you're worried about your pouch moving or getting uncomfortable throughout the day, consider using an ostomy belt or wrap. These clothes offer support, keep the pouch in place, and boost your confidence.
- Adaptive clothes: Many businesses now provide adaptive clothes made for people who use medical equipment such as ostomy pouches. These clothing often include concealed pockets or holes that enable you to manage your ostomy discreetly without having to completely undress.

Above all, remember that you're not alone. Many individuals continue to work and study with an ostomy, achieving success and satisfaction while adjusting to their new situation. You may flourish in your everyday life with assistance from your workplace or school, as well as a proactive attitude to ostomy management.

Part 7: Relationship and Intimacy

Communicating with Partners: Starting the Conversation about Your Ostomy

Navigating relationships and intimacy with an ostomy may be challenging, but open communication is essential. Many people are afraid to discuss an ostomy with their spouse because of worries about how it may affect intimacy, feelings of rejection, and coping with body image problems. However, beginning this discussion is a vital step toward increasing understanding, emotional support, and preserving intimacy in your relationship.

How to Begin the Conversation about Your Ostomy

Discussing your ostomy with your spouse may seem awkward at first, particularly if you're in the early stages of your relationship or are still adapting to life with a stoma. However, by approaching the issue deliberately, you may create an open and supportive discourse that strengthens your relationship. Here are a few suggestions on how to start:

1. Select the Appropriate Time and Place

Choose a moment when both you and your spouse are calm and not distracted by work or other responsibilities. This chat works best in a calm, private setting where you may both feel comfortable sharing your views and worries. Avoid initiating the talk when emotions are already high, such as during a fight or a hard day.

Some people believe that the greatest moment to disclose an ostomy is when you start talking about other personal or health-related issues. Others may find it simpler to discuss it early on in the relationship, before intimacy becomes an issue. There is no one appropriate moment to bring it up; what matters most is that you are emotionally prepared and in a setting where the talk may take place without pressure or judgment.

2. Be honest and clear

When discussing your ostomy, be as direct as possible. This does not need you to go into graphic detail straight once, but clarity is essential for ensuring your spouse understands the problem. Begin by explaining that your ostomy is caused by a medical ailment or surgery and that you must wear a pouch that collects waste from your body.

You may say something like:

"I'd like to discuss something significant with you. I've undergone surgery that required an ostomy. This means I wear a pouch to assist control my body's waste. It's something I've come to accept, but I wanted to discuss it with you because I value honesty in our relationship.

This style of explanation keeps the discussion focused on facts while yet leaving room for any inquiries your partner may have. If they're unfamiliar with ostomies, be prepared to answer some basic questions about what they are and how they function.

3. Recognize their feelings

Your spouse may be concerned or unclear about how to react, particularly if they are inexperienced with ostomies. It's important to recognize that they may need some time to comprehend the information, and you may welcome them to ask any questions they have. Let them know it's alright to be concerned, and reassure them that their emotions are genuine.

For example:

"I recognize that this is new to you, and you are welcome to ask questions or express concerns. I'm willing to discuss whatever you're concerned about, and we can work things out together."

This method demonstrates empathy and encourages deeper discourse, enabling your partner to express themselves without feeling pressured. Encourage children to express their sentiments, even if they are difficult to understand at first. This is a process that both of you will go through together, and their emotional responses are part of it.

4. Share Your Feelings about Your Ostomy

While this chat is intended to assist your spouse understand your ostomy, it also allows you to communicate how you feel about it. Whether you're feeling confident, worried, or self-conscious, communicating your feelings allows your partner to better comprehend your situation. If you're still adapting, explain that you're processing your emotions and that it may take some time to feel entirely at ease.

For example:

"I am still learning to live with my ostomy, and it has not always been easy. Some days I feel confident, while others I feel self-conscious. But what matters most to me is that we can have open discussions about it and find out how to make things work in our relationship.

Being vulnerable with your emotions may foster closeness and trust, demonstrating to your spouse that you are prepared to be open and honest with them about this important aspect of your life.

Addressing Concerns and Questions

Once you've informed your spouse about your ostomy, he or she will most likely have questions, both practical and emotional. It is critical to be patient and understanding as they digest this new knowledge, as well as to respond to their concerns in a straightforward and deliberate manner.

1. Common Questions Your Partner May Ask

When partners first hear about an ostomy, they often ask similar questions. The following are some of the most prevalent problems, along with suggestions on how to address them.

"Will it change our intimacy?" It's reasonable for your spouse to be concerned about how your ostomy can affect physical intimacy. Reassure them that, although things may be different, you can still enjoy intimacy and have a good relationship. Explain that with some modifications and conversation, many couples discover that their love life remains just as strong. You may say:

"I realize you're worried about closeness; I was too at first. However, I've discovered that it is possible to have a loving and personal relationship with an ostomy. We may need to make some changes, but it does not have to affect how we communicate."

"Will I hurt you if we're intimate?" Your spouse may be concerned about inflicting agony or suffering during intimate times. Reassure them that with proper care and communication, they have no cause to be afraid of injuring you. Inform them that you will communicate if anything makes them uncomfortable, and that, like in any relationship, it is all about finding what works best for both of you.

"I understand that having an ostomy might make things more challenging, but I'll let you know if anything makes you uncomfortable. We can always take things gently, and I'll be honest with you if I need to change anything."

"Will I notice it or feel it during intimacy?" Your spouse may be wondering whether they will feel or detect the pouch during physical contact. You may reassure them that, although the pouch is there, it does not have to be the center of your private times. In fact, many persons with ostomies prefer to wear tiny, unobtrusive pouches or coverings, which make them feel more comfortable and lessen the likelihood of the pouch being discovered.

"You will probably not notice it during intimacy. I have little, discrete bags to utilize, as well as coverings to make it more comfortable for both of us."

2. How to Navigate Concerns Together

Addressing your partner's worries and inquiries with kindness and honesty is essential for sustaining a solid, supportive relationship. Here are a few more suggestions to assist you handle this topic.

- Encourage Open Dialogue: Ensure that your spouse feels comfortable asking follow-up questions or addressing any lingering issues. Tell them that it's appropriate to discuss the ostomy anytime they're hesitant or need reassurance.
- Concentrate on Reassurance and Support: Your spouse may require reassurance that your ostomy does not affect how you feel about them or your relationship. Affirm your emotional connection and thank them for their understanding.

- Normalize the Experience: Point out that many individuals' live full lives with an ostomy, including maintaining healthy and loving relationships. If it seems right, tell anecdotes of other ostomates who have achieved success in their own life to assist normalize the situation.
- Talk about Practical Adjustments**: While emotional concerns are essential, it is also beneficial to address any practical changes you may need to make during intimacy. This might include experimenting with various settings, utilizing pouch covers, or scheduling time to clean and prepare ahead of time.

Above all, be gentle to yourself as you go through these topics. It's normal to feel vulnerable when discussing such intimate details about your life, but open communication can eventually deepen your bond and help you maintain a satisfying, loving relationship with your spouse.

Sexual intimacy and ostomies

Living with an ostomy has unique obstacles, but it does not exclude you from having a satisfying and healthy sexual life. Many persons with ostomies may effectively participate in romantic relationships and become closer to their spouses. Maintaining intimacy with an ostomy requires communication, planning, and self-confidence.

Physical considerations during intimacy

When it comes to intimacy, your body may feel different following ostomy surgery, but this does not rule out sexual activity. You may need to make changes to feel more comfortable, and your partner will most likely welcome advice on what works best for you. Many individuals with ostomies continue to have gratifying and pleasant sex lives, but it's vital to understand how the operation affects your body and what physical changes you could notice.

1. **Energy and comfort**

Depending on the sort of surgery you had, you may feel tired or sensitive in the first stages of recuperation. Allow yourself time to recover before participating in sexual activity. The healing process varies depending on the kind of ostomy, but it might take many weeks to months before you are ready for intimacy.

Even after your body has physically recovered, you may still feel uncomfortable or hesitant to do certain motions. You'll need to discover the most comfortable postures for you and avoid putting pressure on the stoma site. For some patients, trying with various postures might help to reduce their pain. Communication with your partner is essential here; tell them if you need to go slower or attempt a different position.

2. Sensitivity and Nerve Alterations

Depending on the kind of surgery you have, you may notice changes in sensation in your abdomen or pelvis. Some individuals report feeling less sensitive at their stoma, while others may have heightened sensitivity in that area. If your operation impacted nerves in the pelvis, it might impede your sexual response or capacity to orgasm. If you detect any changes in your sexual function, contact your healthcare physician right away. They may be able to suggest techniques or therapies to help you cope.

Women who have had ostomies may also experience changes in vaginal lubrication or pain during intercourse. If you have vaginal dryness, water-based lubricants might help make intimacy more pleasant. Listen to your body and make modifications that promote your comfort and enjoyment.

Using Products Like Ostomy Wraps or Pouch Covers for Confidence

Body image is one of the most common worries that persons with ostomies have about intimacy. You may be self-conscious about your stoma or pouch, concerned about how it looks or how your spouse may respond. These sentiments are entirely natural, but keep in mind that you have the right to be confident and happy in your own skin.

1. Ostomy Wraps and Belts

Ostomy wraps and belts are intended to provide extra support and security for your ostomy pouch. They may assist hide the pouch, making it more inconspicuous and reducing any noise or movement during intercourse. Many patients find that wearing an ostomy wrap boosts their confidence and makes them less concerned about their pouch being discovered.

Ostomy wraps are normally constructed of soft, elastic fabric that is easy to wear and does not irritate the skin. They come in a number of forms, ranging from basic bands to more ornate outfits, and may be worn beneath clothes or on their own during private times. These wraps also offer rigidity to the pouch, lowering the likelihood of leaks and irritation.

2 Pouch Covers

Pouch coverings are another excellent choice for those who wish to feel more confident during intimate moments. These coverings slide over your ostomy pouch, hiding it and improving its look. Pouch covers come in a range of fabrics and colors, so you may select one that feels perfect for you. They may also assist lessen the sound of the bag during movement, giving you more peace of mind.

Using an ostomy wrap or pouch cover is a simple approach to recover confidence and concentrate on your relationship with your spouse rather than the pouch's look or movement. It may help you transition from self-consciousness to empowerment by reminding you that your ostomy does not determine your value or beauty.

3. Communicate with Your Partner

Confidence is strongly linked to how you feel in your relationship. Open and honest chats with your spouse about your worries may help ease much of the anxiety associated with intimacy. If you're concerned about how the pouch may affect your sexual experience, discuss your worries with your partner and work together to find solutions. Wearing an ostomy wrap or pouch cover is one option that might help both of you feel more at ease and enjoy the event without distractions.

Pregnancy and Fertility Considerations for Men and Women with Ostomies

Many individuals with ostomies have concerns regarding fertility, pregnancy, and their ability to have children after surgery. It is crucial to understand that, in most situations, having an ostomy does not exclude you from having children, but there are certain unique concerns for both men and women.

1. Women with Ostomies

Many ostomies result in healthy pregnancies and deliveries. However, pregnancy with an ostomy might provide particular complications. First and foremost, when contemplating a pregnancy, talk with your healthcare team so that they can advise you on how to manage your ostomy throughout pregnancy and address any surgery-related problems.

Here are some key aspects to consider:

- Stoma Size and Location: As your abdomen expands during pregnancy, your stoma may alter size or form. The position of your stoma may also change as your abdomen grows. It is critical to regularly monitor your stoma throughout pregnancy and collaborate with your ostomy nurse or doctor to make any required changes to your ostomy equipment.
- Pouching Changes: During pregnancy, you may need to modify your ostomy pouch, particularly if your stoma grows or moves. Regular visits to your healthcare practitioner can assist ensure that you use the most comfortable and effective items throughout your pregnancy.
- Monitoring Hydration and Nutrition: It is critical to stay hydrated and eat well throughout pregnancy, especially if you have an ileostomy. Your healthcare practitioner may advise you on how to keep a balanced diet and remain hydrated, all of which are critical for your and your baby's health.
- Labor and Delivery: Many women with ostomies may have vaginal births. However, in rare situations, a C-section may be required, particularly if your operation affected the pelvic region or if there are any worries about the strain on your stoma during delivery. To ensure a safe and easy birth, you should explore delivery alternatives with your obstetrician and healthcare team ahead of time.

2. Men with Ostomies

For males, ostomy surgery may occasionally compromise fertility, especially if the procedure included the pelvic region or if nerves connected to sexual function were damaged. Some men may have trouble with erections or ejaculation after surgery, which might impair their ability to conceive naturally. However, many men with ostomies may still father children, and there are reproductive treatments and medical choices available for those who are having difficulty.

If you are worried about your fertility following ostomy surgery, see an urologist or fertility expert. They can evaluate your circumstances and provide solutions for maintaining or improving fertility. In certain circumstances, sperm retrieval or assisted reproductive technologies (ART) such as in vitro fertilization (IVF) may be used.

Sexual intimacy with an ostomy is a very personal experience that may need changes and obstacles, but keep in mind that your ostomy does not affect your value, beauty, or capacity to have a meaningful sex life. There are several methods to enjoy intimacy and establish a healthy, loving relationship, including trying various positions, wearing ostomy covers to boost confidence, and talking through difficulties with your spouse.

For individuals contemplating motherhood, having an ostomy does not stop them from having children. With adequate preparation, healthcare assistance, and self-care, many persons with ostomies may have successful pregnancies and children.

Finally, the most crucial component of intimacy—whether sexual, emotional, or relational—is the connection you have with your partner. You may keep a strong, intimate relationship going by concentrating on open discussion, mutual understanding, and shared experiences.

Part 8: Long-Term Health and Ostomy Maintenance

Maintaining long-term health for people with ostomies requires continual care and attention to both their physical well-being and the ostomy site. While you may ultimately acquire used to daily care routines, it's vital to remember that regular medical check-ups and expert supervision are necessary to ensure the health of your stoma and general wellbeing.

Regular Medical Check-Ups: The Key to Long-Term Ostomy Care

Following your first recuperation from ostomy surgery, you may feel comfortable maintaining your stoma on your own. However, frequent check-ins with your healthcare practitioner, especially your WOC nurse, are essential for monitoring both the health of your stoma and your general wellness. Even if everything seems to be in order, regular check-ups might detect problems before they worsen.

1. How Often Should You See Your Doctor or WOC Nurse?

The frequency of medical check-ups will depend on your specific circumstances, the kind of ostomy you have, and any underlying health concerns that may affect your treatment. However, some broad recommendations might help you decide when to schedule these consultations.

- Initial Post-Surgery Period: During the weeks after ostomy surgery, you will most likely need more regular visits to your WOC nurse. These checkups will assist ensure that your stoma heals effectively, that you are utilizing the appropriate ostomy equipment, and that any possible issues are identified early on. Follow-up appointments are usually scheduled within a week or two after surgery, as well as one month and three months afterward.
- One Year of Ostomy Care: It is advised that you see your WOC nurse or doctor every few months for check-ups throughout the first

year following surgery. These visits are critical for altering your ostomy care regimen, evaluating the skin surrounding your stoma, and ensuring that you are correctly managing your nutrition and hydration. Your nurse may also evaluate your mental and emotional well-being, since adapting to life with an ostomy may take time.
- Ongoing Long-Term Care: After the first year, your visits may be reduced to every six months or once a year, depending on your health and any difficulties you may encounter. During these appointments, your WOC nurse will check your stoma for changes in size, shape, or color. They will also inspect the skin surrounding the stoma for symptoms of irritation or infection, as well as confirm that your appliances continue to fit correctly. If you are suffering leakage, pain, or irritation, you may need to schedule more regular appointments until the problem is fixed.

2. When to Get Immediate Medical Attention

In addition to periodic check-ups, there are several circumstances in which you should seek emergency medical attention, even if you do not have a planned appointment. This includes:

- Changes in Stoma Appearance**: If your stoma changes color (e.g., pale, purple, or black), grows in size abruptly, or retracts into the belly, it may indicate a major problem. Changes in appearance may signal issues with blood flow, hernias, or stoma retraction, all of which need rapid medical attention.

- Frequent Leaks or Appliance Issues: If you have frequent leaks or your ostomy pouch no longer fits securely, you should visit with your WOC nurse. Leaks may cause skin irritation or infection if not handled promptly. Your nurse may assist you change your appliance's fit or propose other goods.

- Discomfort or Discomfort around the Stoma: While some sensitivity around the stoma is typical, persistent discomfort, tenderness, or swelling may signal an infection or other problem. If you encounter these symptoms, particularly if they are accompanied by fever or redness, get medical assistance right once.

- Dehydration or Digestive Issues: If you have an ileostomy or colostomy and observe symptoms of dehydration (such as dry mouth, dizziness, or reduced urine output), or if you have severe diarrhea, you should visit your doctor. Ostomates are more susceptible to dehydration, and continuing digestive difficulties may need dietary changes or further medical intervention.

When to Consider Revision Surgery or Reversal

Ostomy surgery may be life-changing, bringing relief from diseases such as intestinal disease, cancer, or serious injuries. However, over time, some people may have difficulties or lifestyle changes that prompt them to contemplate revision procedures or, in some situations, ostomy reversal. These operations may be complicated and based on your individual medical circumstances, so it's important to explore the risks and advantages with your doctor.

1. When and Why Revision Surgery May Be Necessary

Ostomy revision surgery is any technique that aims to amend or repair an existing ostomy. These procedures may be necessary owing to stoma difficulties, changes in your anatomy, or problems with your ostomy equipment. The following are some frequent reasons why revision surgery may be recommended:

- Stoma Prolapse: A prolapsed stoma occurs when the intestine flexes outward through the stoma, causing it to stretch more than normal. While modest prolapse may be treated without surgery, severe instances may need surgical intervention to avoid pain or consequences.
- Stoma Retraction: In certain situations, the stoma retracts or sinks below the skin's surface, making it difficult to properly connect ostomy equipment. This may cause leaks, skin irritation, and infections. Surgery may be required to relocate the stoma and avoid future issues.
- Parastomal Hernia: A parastomal hernia develops when a portion of the intestine protrudes through the abdominal wall near the stoma. This might generate a protrusion under the skin, causing pain. In

certain circumstances, surgery may be necessary to correct the hernia and strengthen the abdominal wall.

- Θ Persistent Skin Irritation: If you continue to have skin irritation or infections after using various ostomy equipment and skin care regimens, surgery to change the size or placement of your stoma may be recommended.

2. Is Ostomy Reversal an Option for You?

For some people, ostomy surgery is just temporary and may be reversed after the underlying problem has cured or improved. Ostomy reversal includes reconnecting the intestines and sealing the stoma, enabling the patient to restore normal bowel function. However, ostomy reversal is not a possibility for everyone, and the choice to pursue it is based on various variables.

- Type of Ostomy: Not all ostomies can be reversed. Ileostomies and colostomies may be reversed if the underlying problem (such as diverticulitis or inflammatory bowel disease) has improved or gone into remission. Urostomies, which redirect urine, are often permanent and cannot be reversed.
- Intestinal Health: For reversal surgery to be effective, the remaining parts of the intestine must be healthy and capable of returning to normal digestive activities. If the intestines have been severely damaged or big parts have been removed during surgery, reversal may be impossible.
- Issues and Risk Factors**: Any issues you've had with your ostomy may affect your choice to reverse it. For example, if you have extensive scar tissue (adhesions) or have had previous procedures, the hazards of reversal surgery may exceed the benefits. Furthermore, those with certain health issues, such as heart disease or diabetes, may be more vulnerable during surgery.
- Recovery and Lifestyle Factors: It's critical to remember that ostomy reversal is a serious procedure with its own dangers and recovery time. You should be prepared for any digestive difficulties, such as diarrhea or constipation, after the reversal. For some people, the benefits of having an ostomy outweigh the risks of not having one. A detailed conversation with your physician and surgeon is required to establish the best course of action

Encouragement and Final Advice: Embracing Life beyond the Ostomy

As you near the conclusion of this guide, take a moment to reflect on the trip you've taken—not only via the pages of this book, but also in your own life. Living with an ostomy may not be something you ever anticipated for yourself, yet here you are, demonstrating perseverance, fortitude, and flexibility on a daily basis.

Your ostomy is neither a restriction nor an impediment to living completely and freely. In reality, for many, it is a gateway to a higher quality of life—free of the pain, disease, or condition that prompted the surgery in the first place. It's tempting to focus on the obstacles, which are genuine, yet there is a new chapter in your life. One that is full of promise, opportunity, and the freedom to live your life on your own.

Having an ostomy does not spell the end of life. It may vary, develop, and offer new learning curves, but it persists—and often grows richer and more meaningful as you adapt and conquer. This book covers everything from the practical elements of ostomy care to managing relationships, employment, travel, and fitness. These chapters cover not just how to manage the technical parts of your ostomy, but also how to flourish, recover confidence, and live a full life despite the changes.

Whether your ostomy is permanent or temporary, it is just part of your tale, not the whole one. There is life after the ostomy—a life full of pleasure, satisfaction, and purpose. Your ostomy does not define you; rather, it shapes the way you live, love, and move ahead.

It is normal to mourn the life you had before surgery. Change is never easy, and adapting to life with an ostomy requires time, tolerance, and compassion for oneself. But once you find your rhythm, you'll realize that your new normal isn't something to dread, but rather something to enjoy. The practical recommendations, guidance, and methods in this book are intended to help you through this new chapter, but they are just tools. The true change takes place inside you, as you choose to embrace your body, respect your path, and go ahead with grace and confidence.

This new normal may not look like what you imagined, but it is up to you to mold it. Every day, you'll get stronger, more comfortable, and at ease with the changes. Do not hasten the procedure. Celebrate your successes, no matter how minor they may seem. Every moment of self-care, every successful adjustment, and every discussion in which you felt heard and understood—it's all part of your journey.

You may feel everything—frustration, appreciation, hope, and struggle—but remember how far you've come. You are characterized not by your challenges, but by how you conquer them.

As you CLOSE this book, take a time to consider how far you've come. Living with an ostomy may not have been your ideal route, but it has brought you to a place of resilience and strength. There is thankfulness in that—deep, profound appreciation for your body's capacity to adapt, for the assistance you've received, and for your own fortitude in confronting this challenge.

Remember to be gentle to yourself, even on difficult days. Allow yourself to celebrate your progress and believe that there is more ahead of you. Your ostomy is not the end of your adventure; rather, it marks a fresh beginning. With each step, you begin a new chapter in your life—one full of possibility, progress, and the promise of what is to come.

Thank you for believing in your own power and the possibilities of what lies ahead. There is so much that awaits you, including new experiences, relationships, and chances to live completely. Your future is bright, and it is yours to shape.

So here's to life after the ostomy. Here's to accepting your new normal with open arms and an open heart. Here's to the trip ahead and the strength you've shown along the way.

You've got it.

Glossary of Terms

- Adhesive: A sticky adhesive used to connect the ostomy equipment to the skin.
- Barrier: A protective covering between the skin and the ostomy equipment to avoid irritation.
- Colostomy: A surgical technique where a portion of the colon is rerouted to a stoma on the abdomen.
- Convexity: A characteristic in certain ostomy barriers that helps the device fit better to avoid leaks, especially for recessed or flat stomachs.
- Dehydration: A condition that develops when the body loses more fluids than it takes in, which is prevalent in patients with an ileostomy.
- Electrolyte imbalance: A disturbance in the equilibrium of electrolytes, such as sodium and potassium, which may develop in persons with certain kinds of ostomies.
- Flange: The component of a two-piece ostomy system that joins the bag to the barrier or baseplate.
- Hernia: A bulge or protrusion of an organ through the muscle or tissue that ordinarily confines it. In the case of ostomy patients, a **parastomal hernia** may occur around the stoma.
- Ileostomy: A surgical technique in which the small intestine is brought through the abdominal wall to establish a stoma.
- Loop stoma: A stoma when a loop of the bowel is brought to the surface of the abdomen and is typically transitory.
- One-piece system: A form of ostomy device where the barrier and the pouch are united in one piece.
- Peristomal skin: The patch of skin surrounding the stoma.
- Prolapsed stoma: When a piece of the bowel telescopes out of the stoma, making it longer than normal.
- Retracted stoma: When the stoma pushes back into the abdomen, typically leading to concerns with appliance adherence and leakage.
- Skin barrier: A product that shields the skin from injury caused by the ostomy output or sticky materials.

- Stoma: The orifice on the abdomen produced after ostomy surgery, through which waste is conveyed.
- Two-piece system: An ostomy appliance system where the barrier and pouch are separate and may be removed and reattached.
- WOC Nurse: Wound, Ostomy, and Continence Nurse. A skilled healthcare practitioner who aids in the treatment of patients with ostomies.

Common Medical Codes and Insurance Tips

Common Medical Codes (U.S.): These codes assist in identifying the medical need of ostomy products and treatments. Below are some of the important codes you may need:

ICD-10 Codes (International Classification of Diseases, 10th Edition):

- Z93.3: Colostomy status - Z93.2: Ileostomy status - Z93.6: Urostomy status - **CPT Codes** (Current Procedural Terminology):
- 44146: Colostomy, including construction and correction
- 44310: Ileostomy, including construction and correction
- 50715: Urostomy procedure

HCPCS Codes (Healthcare Common Procedure Coding System): These codes are used to charge for ostomy products.

- A4388: Ostomy pouch, two-piece system, closed
- A4390: Ostomy pouch, one-piece system, drainable
- A4361: Ostomy faceplate or barrier, with flange (two-piece system)

Insurance Tips for Ostomy Supplies:

- Know Your Plan: Before buying ostomy supplies, research your insurance plan to understand what is covered. Some plans demand prior clearance for specific goods.
- Ask about Allowable Quantities: Many insurance companies have restrictions on the amount of ostomy supplies (pouches, barriers, etc.) they will cover during a set period. Be careful to specify this to prevent unwanted fees.
- Out-of-Pocket Costs: Understand your co-pays, deductibles, and any out-of-pocket maximums for ostomy-related treatment and supplies.

- Durable Medical Equipment (DME) Providers: Ostomy supplies are typically designated Durable Medical Equipment. Ask your insurance carrier for a list of authorized DME vendors.
- Appeals Process: If a claim is refused, don't hesitate to challenge the decision. This is frequently effective if you produce proof from your healthcare practitioner concerning the medical need of your products.

List of National and International Ostomy Support Organizations

United States:

- United Ostomy Associations of America (UOAA): [www.ostomy.org] (https://www.ostomy.org); The UOAA offers a multitude of resources, including instructional materials, a list of support groups, and advocacy information.
- Crohn's & Colitis Foundation: [www.crohnscolitisfoundation.org] (https://www.crohnscolitisfoundation.org) - For those with IBD, this foundation provides support, education, and research updates.
- Wound, Ostomy, and Continence Nurses Society (WOCN): [www.wocn.org] (https://www.wocn.org); This association offers assistance and resources for patients and professionals, including how to identify a local WOC nurse.

United Kingdom

- Colostomy UK: [www.colostomyuk.org] (https://www.colostomyuk.org) - This charity offers support, education, and guidance for individuals with colostomies, as well as information on living with a stoma.
- Ileostomy and Internal Pouch Association (IA): [www.iasupport.org] (https://www.iasupport.org) - IA provides support for persons living with an ileostomy or internal pouch, with access to an assistance network and hotline.

Canada

- Ostomy Canada Society: [www.ostomycanada.ca] (https://www.ostomycanada.ca); Ostomy Canada offers help for Canadians with ostomies and their families, giving a support network and education resources.

Australia

Ostomy Association of Australia**: [www.ostomysa.org.au] (https://www.ostomysa.org.au); this organization offers services, support, and product information to ostomates in Australia.

International

International Ostomy Association (IOA): [www.ostomyinternational.org] (https://www.ostomyinternational.org) - The IOA is a worldwide organization that unites ostomy groups from across the globe, delivering assistance and advocacy at an international level.

Manufacturers and Suppliers of Ostomy Products

- Hollister Incorporated: [www.hollister.com] (https://www.hollister.com) - Hollister manufactures a comprehensive variety of ostomy products, including pouches, skin barriers, and accessories. Their goods are regarded for comfort and security.
- Coloplast: [www.coloplast.us] (https://www.coloplast.us) - Coloplast provides a variety of ostomy care solutions, including one- and two-piece systems, skin barriers, and protective accessories.
- ConvaTec: [www.convatec.com] (https://www.convatec.com) - ConvaTec is a worldwide corporation selling ostomy pouches, adhesives, and other solutions that attempt to increase comfort and reduce leakage.
- B. Braun: [www.bbraun.com] (https://www.bbraun.com) - B. Braun offers a range of ostomy care items, from pouches to skin barriers, emphasizing on cleanliness and convenience of use.
- Securi-T USA: www.securitusa.com Specializing in economical ostomy products, Securi-T USA provides a choice of trustworthy pouches and attachments that focus cost-effectiveness without compromising quality. .

Printed in Great Britain
by Amazon